Procedure Checklists for Craven and Hirnle's

Fundamentals of Nursing

HUMAN HEALTH AND FUNCTION

SIXTH EDITION

Procedure Checklists for Craven and Hirnle's

Fundamentals of Nursing

HUMAN HEALTH AND FUNCTION

SIXTH EDITION

Ruth F. Craven, EdD, RN, FAAN

Constance J. Hirnle, MN, RN

Wolters Kluwer | Lippincott Williams & Wilkins
Health
Philadelphia · Baltimore · New York · London
Buenos Aires · Hong Kong · Sydney · Tokyo

Executive Editor: Jean Rodenberger
Senior Production Editor: Marian A. Bellus
Director of Nursing Production: Helen Ewan
Managing Editor / Production: Erika Kors
Art Director, Design: Joan Wendt
Art Director, Illustration: Brett MacNaughton
Manufacturing Coordinator: Karin Duffield
Compositor: Circle Graphics
Printer: Victor Graphics

6th Edition

9 8 7 6 5 4 3 2 1

ISBN: 978-0-7817-8024-7

Printed in the United States of America

Care has been taken to confirm the accuracy of the information presented and to describe generally accepted practices. However, the authors, editors, and publisher are not responsible for errors or omissions or for any consequences from application of the information in this book and make no warranty, expressed or implied, with respect to the currency, completeness, or accuracy of the contents of the publication. Application of this information in a particular situation remains the professional responsibility of the practitioner; the clinical treatments described and recommended may not be considered absolute and universal recommendations.

The authors, editors, and publisher have exerted every effort to ensure that drug selection and dosage set forth in this text are in accordance with the current recommendations and practice at the time of publication. However, in view of ongoing research, changes in government regulations, and the constant flow of information relating to drug therapy and drug reactions, the reader is urged to check the package insert for each drug for any change in indications and dosage and for added warnings and precautions. This is particularly important when the recommended agent is a new or infrequently employed drug.

Some drugs and medical devices presented in this publication have Food and Drug Administration (FDA) clearance for limited use in restricted research settings. It is the responsibility of the health care provider to ascertain the FDA status of each drug or device planned for use in his or her clinical practice.

Contents

Name _____ Date _____

Unit _____ Position _____

Instructor/Evaluator: _____ Position _____

PROCEDURE 25-1
Measuring Weight

Goal: To provide baseline data from which to assess total fluid balance or nutritional status; to provide baseline data to determine drug dosages or information for diagnostic testing with dye or radioactive injections.

Excellent	Satisfactory	Needs Practice		Comments
____	____	____	1. Have client void before weighing.	
____	____	____	2. Use the same scale and measure the weight at the same time each day. Client should wear same clothing for each weight measurement. He or she should remove slippers or shoes before measurement.	
____	____	____	3. Place protective paper or cloth on scale.	
____	____	____	4. Check that scale registers zero. Adjust as necessary.	

Weight With Standing Scale

____	____	____	1. Assist client onto scale. Client must stand in center of platform and not lean or hold onto supports.	
____	____	____	2. Read digital display or adjust counterweights to determine client's weight.	
____	____	____	3. Assist client from scale and record weight in the client's record.	

Weight With Chair Scale

____	____	____	1. Place scale beside client and lock wheels.	
____	____	____	2. Transfer client onto chair. If arm of chair is removable, unlock and remove before transfer. Lock back into place after transfer.	
____	____	____	3. Read digital display or adjust counterweights to determine client's weight.	
____	____	____	4. Transfer client back to bed or wheelchair.	
____	____	____	5. Clean the scale according to agency policy. Return to proper location and plug in.	

Weight With Bed Scale

____	____	____	1. Elevate client's bed to level of stretcher scale.	
____	____	____	2. With one or two assistants, turn client on the side with back toward the scale.	
____	____	____	3. Roll scale toward the bed, lock wheels in place, and lower stretcher onto bed.	
____	____	____	4. Position folded stretcher under client. Roll client onto stretcher.	

PROCEDURE 25-1
Measuring Weight (*Continued*)

Excellent	Satisfactory	Needs Practice		Comments
			Goal: To provide baseline data from which to assess total fluid balance or nutritional status; to provide baseline data to determine drug dosages or information for diagnostic testing with dye or radioactive injections.	
____	____	____	5. Attach stretcher arms to stretcher and gradually elevate stretcher about 2 inches above mattress surface. Inform client before elevating. Reassure the client that he or she will not fall but the head may feel lower than the body.	
____	____	____	6. Determine that the stretcher is not touching any equipment. Lift all drains and tubing away from stretcher.	
____	____	____	7. Read digital display for client's weight. *Note:* This is a good time to change client's linen as he or she is elevated off the bed.	
____	____	____	8. Gradually lower stretcher to the bed. Remove stretcher arms and transfer client off stretcher. Remove stretcher.	
____	____	____	9. Unlock bed scale wheels and move away from bed.	
____	____	____	10. Assist client to comfortable position.	
____	____	____	11. Clean stretcher and scale according to agency policy. Return to proper location and keep plugged in for next use.	
____	____	____	12. Record weight, and note any extra linen or equipment weighed with the client.	

Procedure Checklists for Craven and Hirnle's Fundamentals of Nursing: Human Health and Function, 6th edition

Name _____   Date _____

Unit _____   Position _____

Instructor/Evaluator: _____   Position _____

Excellent	Satisfactory	Needs Practice	PROCEDURE 25-2 **Assessing the Neurologic System**	Comments
			Goal: To obtain baseline information about the client's neurologic status; to assess the client's orientation to his or her environment; to evaluate the client's cognitive function and ability to make judgments; to assess the integrity of motor and sensory pathways and the client's ability to ambulate safely; to detect increased intracranial pressure; to detect changes in neurologic status.	
____ ____ ____			**Cognitive–Sensory Assessment** 1. Assess the client's level of consciousness by asking direct questions that require a verbal response. Note appropriateness of response and emotional state.	
____ ____ ____			2. Evaluate client's speech patterns.	
____ ____ ____			3. Observe general appearance: hygiene, appropriateness of clothing to setting and weather.	
____ ____ ____			4. If client responses are inappropriate, ask direct questions related to person, place, and time (e.g., "What is your name?" "Where are you right now?" "What city do you live in?" "What day is this?").	
____ ____ ____			5. If client doesn't respond or inappropriately responds to orientation questions, give simple commands (e.g., "Squeeze my fingers," "Wiggle your toes"). If the client gives no response to verbal commands, test response to painful stimuli by applying firm pressure on client's sternum or finger nailbed with your thumb.	
____ ____ ____			6. Document cognitive or sensory assessment objectively by stating specific client responses to verbal or tactile stimulation. Use of Glasgow Coma Scale helps charting of frequent level-of-consciousness testing.	
____ ____ ____			7. Assess function of cranial nerves.	
____ ____ ____			8. Assess sensory pathways:	
____ ____ ____			a. Client's eyes are closed during all sensory tests.	
____ ____ ____			b. Apply stimuli to skin in a random, unpredictable order while comparing one side of body with the other.	
____ ____ ____			c. Client should verbally state when he or she feels a particular stimulus. If you detect an area of altered sensation, note which spinal cord segment is affected by referring to a dermatome chart.	

PROCEDURE 25-2
Assessing the Neurologic System (*Continued*)

Goal: To obtain baseline information about the client's neurologic status; to assess the client's orientation to his or her environment; to evaluate the client's cognitive function and ability to make judgments; to assess the integrity of motor and sensory pathways and the client's ability to ambulate safely; to detect increased intracranial pressure; to detect changes in neurologic status.

Excellent	Satisfactory	Needs Practice		Comments
____	____	____	9. Test pain sensation first by lightly touching the pointed, then the blunt, end of sterile toothpick to proximal and distal aspects of the arm and legs.	
____	____	____	10. Test temperature sensation by touching skin with vials of hot, then cold, water.	
____	____	____	11. Lightly stroke proximal and distal aspects of client's arms and legs with a cotton applicator or ball. Ask client to tell you when and where each stroke is felt.	
____	____	____	12. Apply a vibrating tuning fork to the distal interphalangeal joints of fingers and great toe. Ask client to describe what he or she feels and when it stops. *Note:* If client does not feel vibration, move the tuning fork proximally to the next joint until sensation is felt.	
			Activity–Mobility Assessment	
____	____	____	13. Inspect arm and leg muscles for atrophy, tremors, fasciculations, or other abnormal movements.	
____	____	____	14. Assess strength of specific muscle groups by having client extend or flex individual joints against resistance provided by examiner's hands. Test biceps, triceps, wrist, leg muscles, and ankle.	
____	____	____	15. Ask client to close eyes and hold arms in front of body with palms up. Have client hold position for 30 seconds and observe for pronation of hands or drifting of arms (pronator drift). *Note:* Notice weaknesses on one or both sides.	
____	____	____	16. Evaluate coordination and balance	
____	____	____	a. Perform a series of rapid alternating movements.	
____	____	____	(1) Have client pat upper thigh by rapidly alternating his or her palm and back of the hand.	
____	____	____	(2) With dominant hand, have client touch his or her thumb to each finger on that hand as quickly as possible.	
____	____	____	(3) Have client use his or her dominant forefinger to first touch your forefinger, then his or her nose. Instruct client to repeat this many times as fast as he or she can.	

PROCEDURE 25-2
Assessing the Neurologic System (*Continued*)

Excellent	Satisfactory	Needs Practice	**Goal:** To obtain baseline information about the client's neurologic status; to assess the client's orientation to his or her environment; to evaluate the client's cognitive function and ability to make judgments; to assess the integrity of motor and sensory pathways and the client's ability to ambulate safely; to detect increased intracranial pressure; to detect changes in neurologic status.	Comments
____	____	____	b. Romberg test: Ask client to stand with feet together, arms at sides. Have client maintain this position for 30 seconds with eyes open, then 30 seconds with eyes closed. Assess for swaying. Stay close to client to assist in case he or she begins to fall.	
____	____	____	c. Ask client to walk across the room. Observe gait for symmetry, rhythm, limping, shuffling, or other abnormalities.	
____	____	____	17. Assess deep tendon reflexes.	
____	____	____	a. Compare symmetry of reflex on each side of body.	
____	____	____	b. Extremity to be tested should be completely relaxed and slightly extended.	
____	____	____	c. Hold the reflex hammer loosely and allow it to swing freely in an arc.	
____	____	____	d. Tap tendon briskly.	
____	____	____	e. Document reflexes by grading from 0 to 4+ on stickman, comparing bilaterally.	

Procedure Checklists for Craven and Hirnle's Fundamentals of Nursing: Human Health and Function, 6th edition

Name _____ Date _____

Unit _____ Position _____

Instructor/Evaluator: _____ Position _____

PROCEDURE 25-3
Auscultating Heart Sounds

Goal: To assess normal and abnormal functioning of the heart valves; to detect cardiac problems.

Excellent	Satisfactory	Needs Practice		Comments
____	____	____	1. Wash hands.	
____	____	____	2. Assist the client to the supine position for auscultation. You may want to re-examine the client in the upright sitting position and a left lateral position. Lift client's gown to expose the chest.	
____	____	____	3. Warm the diaphragm of the stethoscope by holding it between your hands for a few moments.	
____	____	____	4. Listen in the mitral area using the diaphragm. Identify the first and second heart sounds (S_1 and S_2). Count the heart rate, noting whether the rhythm is regular or irregular. If the rhythm is irregular, count the heart rate for a full minute. Also note whether the irregularity has a pattern or whether it is totally unpredictable.	
____	____	____	5. Listen in the aortic area using the diaphragm. Concentrate first on S_1, then S_2, noting whether splitting occurs. Shift your concentration to systole and then diastole; listen for extra sounds, such as murmurs.	
____	____	____	6. Listen in the pulmonic area, still using only the diaphragm. Repeat the sequence described in step 5, concentrating on S_1, S_2, systole, and diastole. Compare the loudness of S_2 in the aortic and pulmonic areas.	
____	____	____	7. Move the diaphragm and listen to the tricuspid and mitral areas.	
____	____	____	8. Return to the aortic area, this time using the bell of the stethoscope. As before, concentrate individually on S_1, S_2, systole, and diastole.	
____	____	____	9. Repeat the same process, using the bell, in the pulmonic, tricuspid, and mitral areas. Especially in the mitral area, concentrate during diastole to detect the presence of a third or fourth heart sound.	
____	____	____	10. Replace the client's clothes. Assist the client to a comfortable position.	
____	____	____	11. Record your assessment findings, describing the intensity, quality, and location of the sounds.	

Procedure Checklists for Craven and Hirnle's Fundamentals
of Nursing: Human Health and Function, 6th edition

Name _____   Date _____

Unit _____   Position _____

Instructor/Evaluator: _____   Position _____

Excellent	Satisfactory	Needs Practice	PROCEDURE 25-4 **Auscultating Breath Sounds**	Comments
			Goal: To listen for variations in breath sounds that may indicate the presence of airway obstruction or disease process; to assess the effectiveness of medications or therapies in opening or clearing airways; to detect fluid volume excess or pulmonary edema.	
____	____	____	1. Wash hands.	
____	____	____	2. Assist the client to an upright sitting position. Remove client's gown to expose chest.	
____	____	____	3. Warm the diaphragm of the stethoscope by holding it between your hands for a short time.	
____	____	____	4. Ask client to breathe deeply through the mouth. Client should breathe slowly.	
			Auscultate Anterior Chest	
____	____	____	5. Place diaphragm of stethoscope about 1 inch below the middle of the right clavicle, making sure it lies between the ribs. Listen to one full inspiration and exhalation. Repeat the process at the corresponding site on the left side.	
____	____	____	6. Note normal and adventitious breath sounds at each point on the chest as you proceed.	
____	____	____	7. Move stethoscope downward about 1.5 to 2 inches along midclavicular line. Note sounds; move stethoscope laterally to opposite side.	
____	____	____	8. Move stethoscope downward another inch or two along midclavicular line to fifth intercostal space. (This space lies just below the nipple line on men, approximately across from the head of the xiphoid process of the sternum.) Note sounds, then move to same spot on opposite side.	
			Auscultate Posterior Chest	
____	____	____	9. Instruct client to lean forward and cross arms in front.	
____	____	____	10. Begin by auscultating the area about 2 inches below the shoulders and 2 inches to the right of the spine. Note sounds, then move to corresponding point on left.	
____	____	____	11. Move stethoscope directly downward 2 or 2.5 inches; note sounds, then move stethoscope laterally and listen on the right.	

PROCEDURE 25-4
Auscultating Breath Sounds (*Continued*)

Excellent	Satisfactory	Needs Practice		Comments
			Goal: To listen for variations in breath sounds that may indicate the presence of airway obstruction or disease process; to assess the effectiveness of medications or therapies in opening or clearing airways; to detect fluid volume excess or pulmonary edema.	
___ ___ ___			12. Repeat process, moving downward 2 to 2.5 inches; listen to corresponding opposite side.	
___ ___ ___			13. Move stethoscope downward to area just below scapula. Listen on right and left. Listen also to areas laterally along lower rib cage.	
___ ___ ___			14. Replace client's clothes and assist the client to a comfortable position.	
___ ___ ___			15. Discuss your findings with the client.	
___ ___ ___			16. Record assessment findings. Be specific as to description and location of adventitious sounds.	

Procedure Checklists for Craven and Hirnle's Fundamentals of Nursing: Human Health and Function, 6th edition

Name _____   Date _____

Unit _____   Position _____

Instructor/Evaluator: _____   Position _____

Excellent	Satisfactory	Needs Practice	PROCEDURE 25-5 **Auscultating Bowel Sounds**	Comments
			Goal: To determine the presence or absence of intestinal peristalsis.	
____	____	____	1. Wash your hands and warm the stethoscope diaphragm.	
____	____	____	2. Ask the client when he or she last ate.	
____	____	____	3. Have the client urinate before the examination.	
____	____	____	4. Assist the client to a supine position with abdomen exposed.	
____	____	____	5. Visually divide the abdomen into four quadrants using the umbilicus as the central crossing landmark.	
____	____	____	6. Place the stethoscope diaphragm in each of the four quadrants. Listen for pitch, frequency, and duration of bowel sounds at each site.	
____	____	____	7. If you do not hear bowel sounds, listen for 3 to 5 minutes in all quadrants before concluding that they are absent.	
____	____	____	8. Proceed with the rest of the physical examination or cover the client's abdomen and assist him or her to a comfortable position.	
____	____	____	9. Document your findings.	

Procedure Checklists for Craven and Hirnle's Fundamentals of Nursing: Human Health and Function, 6th edition

Name _____   Date _____

Unit _____   Position _____

Instructor/Evaluator: _____   Position _____

Excellent	Satisfactory	Needs Practice	PROCEDURE 26-1 **Assessing Body Temperature**	Comments
			Goal: To obtain baseline temperature data for comparing future measurements; to screen for alterations in temperature; to evaluate temperature response to therapies.	

Assessing Oral Temperature with an Electronic Thermometer

Excellent	Satisfactory	Needs Practice		
____	____	____	1. Wash hands. Identify client and explain the procedure.	
____	____	____	2. Remove electronic thermometer from the battery pack, and remove the temperature probe from the recording unit, noting a digital display of temperature on the screen (usually 34°C or 94°F).	
____	____	____	3. Place the disposable cover over the temperature probe and attach securely. Grasp the base of the probe.	
____	____	____	4. Insert the probe below the client's tongue and into the sublingual pocket of the mouth. Ask the client to close his or her lips around the probe. Hold the probe, supporting it in place.	
____	____	____	5. Wait for a beep (usually 10 to 20 seconds), which indicates the estimated temperature. Watch to see if temperature continues to rise. When the temperature reading stops rising, note the temperature displayed on the unit and remove the probe from the client's mouth.	
____	____	____	6. Hold the probe over a waste container and displace the probe cover by pressing the probe release button.	
____	____	____	7. Return the probe to the storage place within the unit and return the thermometer to the battery pack. Cleanse according to agency policy.	
____	____	____	8. Record temperature on vital sign documentation record. Discuss findings with client if appropriate.	

Assessing Rectal Temperature with an Electronic Thermometer

Excellent	Satisfactory	Needs Practice		
____	____	____	1. Wash hands. Don clean gloves. Identify client and explain procedure.	
____	____	____	2. Close bedroom door or bed curtains. Assist client to Sims' position with upper leg flexed. Expose only anal area.	
____	____	____	3. Remove rectal (red) electronic thermometer from battery pack and extend the temperature probe from the unit, noting a digital display of temperature on the screen.	

PROCEDURE 26-1
Assessing Body Temperature (*Continued*)

Excellent	Satisfactory	Needs Practice		Comments

Goal: To obtain baseline temperature data for comparing future measurements; to screen for alterations in temperature; to evaluate temperature response to therapies.

4. Securely attach the disposable cover over the temperature probe.
5. Apply water-soluble lubricant liberally to thermometer probe tip.
6. Separate client's buttocks with one gloved hand until the anal sphincter is visible.
7. Ask client to take a deep, slow breath. Insert thermometer into anus in direction of umbilicus, 1 inch for a child and 1.5 for an adult. Do not force.
8. Hold the probe in place until machine emits a beep. Obtain reading.
9. Follow steps 6 to 8 in Assessing Oral Temperature With Electronic Thermometer.

Assessing Axillary Temperature with an Electronic Thermometer

1. Follow steps 1 to 3 in Assessing Oral Temperature with Electronic Thermometer.
4. Close bedroom door or unit curtains; assist client to comfortable position, and remove clothing to expose axilla.
5. Place thermometer against middle of axilla; fold client's arm down and place across chest, enclosing thermometer in axillary area.
6. Wait for a beep that indicates the estimated temperature. Watch to see if temperature continues to rise. When it stops, note the temperature displayed on the unit and remove the probe from the client's axilla.
7. Follow steps 6 to 8 in Assessing Oral Temperature with Electronic Thermometer.

Assessing Temperature Using a Tympanic Membrane Thermometer

1. Wash hands. Identify client and explain procedure.
2. Remove tympanic thermometer from recharging base and check that the lens is clean. Attach tympanic probe cover to sensor unit.
3. Insert probe into ear canal, making sure the probe fits snugly. Avoid forcing the probe too deeply into the ear. Pulling the pinna back, up, and out in an adult will straighten the ear canal. Some manufacturers recommend moving the thermometer in a figure-eight pattern. Rotate the probe handle toward the jaw line.

PROCEDURE 26-1
Assessing Body Temperature (*Continued*)

Excellent	Satisfactory	Needs Practice	

Goal: To obtain baseline temperature data for comparing future measurements; to screen for alterations in temperature; to evaluate temperature response to therapies.

Comments

4. Activate the thermometer, and note the temperature readout, which is usually displayed within 2 seconds.
5. Eject sensor probe cover directly into waste container, cleanse according to agency policy, and return tympanic thermometer to base for recharging. Store away from temperature extremes.
6. Record temperature on vital sign documentation record. Discuss findings with client if appropriate.

Assessing Temperature Using a Temporal Artery Thermometer

1. Wash hands. Identify client and explain procedure.
2. Remove thermometer from storage base. If low battery indicator shows, replace battery.
3. Inspect the thermometer lens. If not shiny, clean by first wiping with alcohol, then rinsing with water-dampened swabs. Allow to air dry.
4. Attach disposable cover.
5. Move hair to expose forehead and hairline. Measure only exposed side of forehead. If patient is lying on side, measure "up" side only. If patient is perspiring heavily (diaphoretic), consider alternate method (e.g., oral).
6. Place probe flush against the center of the forehead and depress button. Slowly slide probe straight across forehead to hairline. Keeping button depressed, lift the probe from the forehead and touch it against the neck just behind the earlobe.
7. Release the button and read the recorded temperature within 15 seconds. If repeated measurements are necessary, wait at least 30 seconds.
8. Eject probe cover directly into waste container, cleanse according to agency policy, and return temporal thermometer to storage base. Store away from temperature extremes.
9. Record temperature on vital sign documentation record, indicating "TA" for temporal artery site. Discuss findings with client if appropriate.

Procedure Checklists for Craven and Hirnle's Fundamentals
of Nursing: Human Health and Function, 6th edition

Name _____   Date _____

Unit _____   Position _____

Instructor/Evaluator: _____   Position _____

PROCEDURE 26-2
Obtaining a Pulse

Goal: To obtain a baseline measurement of heart rate and rhythm; to evaluate the heart's response to various therapies and medications; peripheral pulse may be palpated to assess local blood flow to an extremity or to monitor perfusion to an extremity following surgery or diagnostic procedures (cardiac catheterization).

Excellent	Satisfactory	Needs Practice		Comments
			Obtaining a Radial Pulse	
___	___	___	1. Wash hands, identify the client, and explain the procedure.	
___	___	___	2. Position client comfortably with forearm across chest or at side with wrist extended.	
___	___	___	3. Place fingertips of your first two or three fingers along the groove at base of thumb, on client's wrist.	
___	___	___	4. Press against radial artery to obliterate pulse, then gradually release pressure until you feel pulsations; assess for regularity and strength.	
___	___	___	5. If pulse is not easily palpable, use Doppler.	
___	___	___	a. Apply conducting gel to end of probe or to radial site.	
___	___	___	b. Press "on" button and place probe against skin on pulse site. Reposition slightly, using firm pressure, until you hear a pulsating sound.	
___	___	___	6. If pulse is regular, count pulse for 30 seconds, and multiply by two. If pulse is irregular, count for 1 full minute. If irregular pulse is a new finding, assess apical radial rate. Count the initial pulse as zero.	
			Obtaining an Apical Pulse	
___	___	___	1. Wash hands, identify the client, and explain the procedure.	
___	___	___	2. Position client in supine or sitting position with sternum and left chest exposed.	
___	___	___	3. Use an alcohol swab to clean the stethoscope and ear pieces before using.	
___	___	___	4. Warm diaphragm of stethoscope by holding it in the palm of your hand for 5 to 10 seconds.	
___	___	___	5. Locate apex of the client's heart by palpating the space between the fifth and sixth rib (fifth intercostal space) and moving to the left midclavicular line.	
___	___	___	6. Insert the ear pieces of stethoscope into your ears and place diaphragm over apex of client's heart.	

PROCEDURE 26-2
Obtaining a Pulse (*Continued*)

Excellent	Satisfactory	Needs Practice	

Goal: To obtain a baseline measurement of heart rate and rhythm; to evaluate the heart's response to various therapies and medications; peripheral pulse may be palpated to assess local blood flow to an extremity or to monitor perfusion to an extremity following surgery or diagnostic procedures (cardiac catheterization).

Comments

____ ____ ____   7. Assess the heartbeat for regularity and dysrhythmias.

____ ____ ____   8. If rhythm is regular, count the heartbeat for 30 seconds, and multiply by two. Count for 1 full minute if the rhythm is irregular. Count the initial pulse as zero.

____ ____ ____   9. Replace the client's gown and assist the client to return to a comfortable position.

____ ____ ____   10. Share results of assessment with client, if appropriate.

____ ____ ____   11. Document pulse on vital sign record or computerized record. Specify in the documentation that you obtained an apical pulse (e.g., AP).

Procedure Checklists for Craven and Hirnle's Fundamentals of Nursing: Human Health and Function, 6th edition

Name _____   Date _____

Unit _____   Position _____

Instructor/Evaluator: _____   Position _____

Excellent	Satisfactory	Needs Practice	PROCEDURE 26-3 **Assessing Respirations** **Goal:** To assess respiratory status by evaluating rate and quality; to evaluate the influence of medications and therapies on respiration.	Comments
____	____	____	1. Wash hands and identify client.	
____	____	____	2. After or before assessment of pulse, keep your fingers resting on client's wrist and observe or feel the rising and falling of chest with respiration. If client is asleep, you may gently place your hand on the client's chest so you can feel chest movement. Do not explain procedure to client.	
____	____	____	3. When you have observed one complete cycle of inspiration and expiration, and if respiration is regular, look at second hand of watch and count the number of complete cycles in 30 seconds and multiply by 2. In children younger than 2 years or in adults with an irregular rate, count for 1 full minute.	
____	____	____	4. If respirations are shallow and difficult to count, observe at the sternal notch.	
____	____	____	5. Note depth and rhythm of respiratory cycle.	
____	____	____	6. Discuss findings with client and document respiratory rate, depth, rhythm, and character.	

Procedure Checklists for Craven and Hirnle's Fundamentals of Nursing: Human Health and Function, 6th edition

Name _____   Date _____

Unit _____   Position _____

Instructor/Evaluator: _____   Position _____

PROCEDURE 26-4
Obtaining Blood Pressure

Goal: To evaluate the client's hemodynamic status by obtaining information about cardiac output, blood volume, peripheral vascular resistance, and arterial wall elasticity; to obtain baseline measurement of blood pressure; to monitor the hemodynamic response to various therapies or disease conditions; to screen for hypertension.

Excellent	Satisfactory	Needs Practice		Comments
___	___	___	1. Wash hands; identify client; explain procedure to client; assist client to a comfortable position with forearm supported at heart level and palm up.	
___	___	___	2. Expose the upper arm completely.	
___	___	___	3. Wrap deflated cuff snugly around upper arm with center of bladder over brachial artery. Lower border of cuff should be about 2 cm above antecubital space (nearer the antecubital space on an infant).	
___	___	___	4. Palpate brachial or radial artery with fingertips. Close valve on pressure bulb and inflate cuff until pulse disappears. Inflate cuff 30 mm Hg higher. Slowly release valve and note reading when pulse reappears.	
___	___	___	5. Fully deflate cuff, and wait 1 to 2 minutes.	
___	___	___	6. Place stethoscope ear piece in ears. Repalpate the brachial artery and place stethoscope bell or diaphragm over site.	
___	___	___	7. Close bulb valve by turning clockwise. Inflate cuff to 30 mm Hg above reading where brachial pulse disappeared.	
___	___	___	8. Slowly release valve so pressure drops about 2 to 3 mm Hg per second.	
___	___	___	9. Identify manometer reading when first clear Korotkoff sound is heard.	
___	___	___	10. Continue to deflate, and note reading when sound muffles or dampens (fourth Korotkoff) and when it disappears (fifth Korotkoff).	
___	___	___	11. Deflate cuff completely and remove from client's arm.	
___	___	___	12. Record blood pressure. Record systolic (e.g., 130) and diastolic (e.g., 80) in the form 130/80. If three pressures are to be recorded, use the form 130/80/40 (40 is the fifth Korotkoff). Abbreviate RA or LA to indicate right or left arm measurement.	
___	___	___	13. Assist client to comfortable position and discuss findings with client, if appropriate.	

Procedure Checklists for Craven and Hirnle's Fundamentals
of Nursing: Human Health and Function, 6th edition

Name _____   Date _____

Unit _____   Position _____

Instructor/Evaluator: _____   Position _____

<table>
<tr><th>Excellent</th><th>Satisfactory</th><th>Needs Practice</th><th>PROCEDURE 26-5
Assessing for Orthostatic Hypotension

Goal: To assess the compensatory status of the cardio-vascular and autonomic nervous systems to changes in body position; to assess for fluid volume deficit; to assess for the client's safety in getting up and ambulating.</th><th>**Comments**</th></tr>
<tr><td>____</td><td>____</td><td>____</td><td>1. Wash hands. Identify client and explain procedure.
2. Position client supine with head of bed flat for 10 minutes.</td><td></td></tr>
<tr><td>____</td><td>____</td><td>____</td><td>3. Check and record supine blood pressure and pulse. Keep blood pressure cuff attached.</td><td></td></tr>
<tr><td>____</td><td>____</td><td>____</td><td>4. Assist client to a sitting position with legs dangling over the edge of the bed. Wait 2 to 4 minutes and check blood pressure and pulse rate. *Note:* The waiting period is a convenient time to auscultate the client's lung fields.</td><td></td></tr>
<tr><td>____</td><td>____</td><td>____</td><td>5. Assist client to standing position. Wait 2 to 4 minutes and check blood pressure and pulse rate. Be alert to signs and symptoms of dizziness.</td><td></td></tr>
<tr><td>____</td><td>____</td><td>____</td><td>6. Assist the client back to a comfortable position.
7. Record measurements and any symptoms that accompanied the postural change. Report a drop of 25 mm Hg in systolic pressure or a drop of 10 mm Hg in diastolic pressure.</td><td></td></tr>
<tr><td>____</td><td>____</td><td>____</td><td>8. Discuss findings with client, if appropriate.</td><td></td></tr>
</table>

Procedure Checklists for Craven and Hirnle's Fundamentals
of Nursing: Human Health and Function, 6th edition

Name _____ Date _____

Unit _____ Position _____

Instructor/Evaluator: _____ Position _____

Excellent	Satisfactory	Needs Practice	PROCEDURE 27-1 **Handwashing**	Comments
			Goal: To reduce the numbers of resident and transient bacteria on the hands; to prevent transfer of microorganisms from healthcare personnel to the client.	
____	____	____	1. Remove all rings except a plain wedding band. Push watch 4 to 5 inches above wrist.	
____	____	____	2. Turn on the water and adjust temperature to warm. Do not splash water or lean against the wet sink. Faucets may be controlled by your hands or may be operated by knee levers or foot pedals.	
____	____	____	3. Hold hands lower than elbows and thoroughly wet hands and lower arms under running water.	
____	____	____	4. Apply soap and rub palms, wrists, and back of hands firmly with circular movements. Interlace fingers and thumbs, moving hands back and forth. Wash at least 1 inch above the area of contamination. If there is no visible soiling, wash to 1 inch above wrists. Continue using plenty of lather and friction for 15 to 30 seconds on each hand. Timing of scrub may vary depending on purpose of wash and amount of contamination.	
____	____	____	5. Clean under fingernails using fingernails of other hand and additional soap. Use orangewood stick if available.	
____	____	____	6. Rinse hands and wrists thoroughly with hands held lower than forearms.	
____	____	____	7. Dry hands and arms thoroughly with paper towel, wiping from fingertips toward forearm. Discard in proper receptacle.	
____	____	____	8. Turn off water using clean, dry paper towel on faucets.	
____	____	____	9. Apply oil-free lotion, especially if skin is dry.	

Procedure Checklists for Craven and Hirnle's Fundamentals of Nursing: Human Health and Function, 6th edition

Name _____   Date _____

Unit _____   Position _____

Instructor/Evaluator: _____   Position _____

Excellent	Satisfactory	Needs Practice	PROCEDURE 27-2 **Donning and Removal of Personal Protective Equipment (PPE)** **Goal:** To prevent transfer of microorganisms via the contact, droplet, and airborne modes of transmission from one client to another; to prevent transmission of microorganisms to self or clothing during client care.	Comments
			Donning PPE	
___	___	___	1. Wash hands.	
___	___	___	2. Unfold the gown in front of you.	
___	___	___	3. Place your arms through the sleeves and tie at the neck and back.	
___	___	___	4. Place the mask at your lower face, secure around ears and pull down mask to cover below chin and fit the nose area securely. If mask has ties, secure the ties above the ears and around the neck. When wearing glasses, be sure to position the mask edge under the glasses. Make sure the mask fits securely and comfortably.	
___	___	___	5. If splash is anticipated, put on goggles or face shield, making sure they fit securely. Alternatively, a face shield with mask can take the place of the mask and goggles.	
___	___	___	6. Don gloves last so that the cuffs of the gloves fit snugly over the cuffs of the gown.	
			Removing PPE	
___	___	___	1. Remain inside the client's door while removing PPE. All used PPE is considered contaminated regardless if visibly soiled. PPE must never be reused.	
___	___	___	2. To remove gloves: First slide your thumb under the cuff of the glove and pull it inside out off your hand. Continue to hold the discarded glove in the other gloved hand and perform the same removal procedure, turning the glove inside out over the discarded glove. Dispose in appropriate waste container. Wash hands.	
___	___	___	3. To remove goggles or face shield: Hold only the headband or ear pieces. Lift away from the face. Place in designated receptacle for reprocessing or in an appropriate waste container.	

Donning and Removal of Personal Protective Equipment (PPE) (*Continued*)

Excellent	Satisfactory	Needs Practice	**Goal:** To prevent transfer of microorganisms via the contact, droplet, and airborne modes of transmission from one client to another; to prevent transmission of microorganisms to self or clothing during client care.	Comments
____	____	____	4. To remove gown: Untie and pull the gown away from you near the neck, grasping from the inside and avoiding touching the outside. Roll it into a ball, inside out, and keep the sleeves inside the ball. Discard in appropriate waste container.	
____	____	____	5. To remove mask: Hold only by earbands or ties (bottom tie first, then top) and move the mask away from the face. Discard in appropriate waste container.	
____	____	____	6. Wash hands thoroughly with an alcohol-based hand sanitizer unless hands are visibly soiled; if they are, then use soap and warm water. If the client has diarrhea or the norovirus, use soap and water.	

Procedure Checklists for Craven and Hirnle's Fundamentals of Nursing: Human Health and Function, 6th edition

Name _____   Date _____

Unit _____   Position _____

Instructor/Evaluator: _____   Position _____

Excellent	Satisfactory	Needs Practice	PROCEDURE 27-3 **Preparing and Maintaining a Sterile Field** **Goal**: To create an environment to prevent the transfer of microorganisms during sterile procedures; to create an environment that helps ensure the sterility of supplies and equipment during a sterile procedure.	Comments
			Preparing a Sterile Field Using a Commercially Prepared Sterile Kit or Tray	
____	____	____	1. Wash your hands.	
____	____	____	2. Inspect the sterile kit for package integrity, contamination, or moisture.	
____	____	____	3. During the entire procedure, never turn your back on the sterile field or lower your hands below the level of the field.	
____	____	____	4. Remove the sterile drape from the outer wrapper and place the inner drape in the center of the work surface, at or above waist level, with the outer flap facing away from you.	
____	____	____	5. Touching the outside of the flap only, reach around (rather than over) the sterile field to open the flap away from you.	
____	____	____	6. Open the side flaps in the same manner, using the right hand for the right flap and the left hand for the left flap.	
____	____	____	7. Lastly, open the innermost flap that faces you, being careful that it does not touch your clothing or any object.	
			Preparing a Sterile Field Using a Packaged Sterile Drape	
____	____	____	1. Open the outer covering of the drape.	
____	____	____	2. Remove the sterile drape by carefully pinching over the top edge (1 inch) of the two corners so that you are touching only the underneath of the sterile drape (bottom, moisture-proof side). Lift the drape carefully out of the package, holding it away from your body and above your waist and work surface.	
____	____	____	3. Continuing to hold only by the pinched-over corners, allow the drape to unfold away from your body and any other surface.	
____	____	____	4. Position the drape on the work surface with the moisture-proof side down (shiny or blue side). Avoid touching any other surface or object with the drape.	

PROCEDURE 27-3
Preparing and Maintaining a Sterile Field (*Continued*)

Goal: To create an environment to prevent the transfer of microorganisms during sterile procedures; to create an environment that helps ensure the sterility of supplies and equipment during a sterile procedure.

Excellent	Satisfactory	Needs Practice		Comments

Adding Sterile Supplies to the Field

5. Open prepackaged sterile supplies by peeling back the partially sealed edge with both hands or lifting up the unsealed edge, taking care not to touch the supplies with your hands.
6. Hold supplies 10 to 12 inches above the field and allow them to fall to the middle of the sterile field.
7. Add wrapped sterile supplies by grasping the sterile object with one hand and unwrapping the flaps with the other hand.
8. Grasp the corners of the wrapper with the free hand and hold them against the wrist of the other hand while you carefully drop the object onto the middle of the sterile field.

Adding Solutions to a Sterile Field

9. Read the solution label and expiration date. Note any signs of contamination.
10. Remove cap and place it with the inside facing up on a flat surface. Do not touch inside of cap or rim of bottle.
11. If bottle has been opened previously, "lip" it by pouring a small amount of solution into a waste container.
12. Hold bottle 6 inches above container on the sterile field and pour slowly to avoid spills. Label solution.
13. Recap the solution bottle and label it with date and time of opening if the solution is to be reused.
14. Add any additional supplies and don sterile gloves (see Procedure 27-3) before starting the procedure.

*Procedure Checklists for Craven and Hirnle's Fundamentals
of Nursing: Human Health and Function,* 6th edition

Name _____ Date _____

Unit _____ Position _____

Instructor/Evaluator: _____ Position _____

Excellent	Satisfactory	Needs Practice	PROCEDURE 27-4 **Applying and Removing Sterile Gloves**	
			Goal: To prevent transfer of microorganisms from hands to sterile objects or open wounds.	**Comments**
			Applying Gloves	
___	___	___	1. Wash hands.	
___	___	___	2. Remove outside wrapper by peeling apart sides.	
___	___	___	3. Lay inner package on clean, flat surface about waist level. Open wrapper from the outside, keeping gloves on inside surface.	
___	___	___	4. Grasp inside edge of the folded cuff of glove with thumb and first two fingers of your dominant hand. Holding hands above waist, insert your nondominant hand into glove. Leave the cuff folded until the opposite hand is gloved.	
___	___	___	5. Slip gloved hand inside the second gloved cuff still in package and pull over dominant hand, extending the cuff down the arm.	
___	___	___	6. Keeping hands above waist, adjust fingers inside the glove and the glove fit, touching only sterile areas.	
			Removing Gloves	
___	___	___	7. With dominant hand, grasp outer surface of nondominant glove just below thumb. Peel off without touching exposed wrist.	
___	___	___	8. Place ungloved hand under thumb side of second cuff and peel off toward the fingers, holding first glove inside second glove. Discard into appropriate receptacle.	
___	___	___	9. Wash hands.	

Procedure Checklists for Craven and Hirnle's Fundamentals of Nursing: Human Health and Function, 6th edition

Name _____ Date _____

Unit _____ Position _____

Instructor/Evaluator: _____ Position _____

Excellent	Satisfactory	Needs Practice	PROCEDURE 28-1 **Administering Oral Medications** **Goal:** To provide a safe, effective, economical route for administering medications; to provide sustained drug action with minimal discomfort.	Comments
____	____	____	1. Wash hands.	
____	____	____	2. Arrange MAR next to medication supply.	
____	____	____	3. Prepare medications for only one client at a time. Check client allergies before removing any medications.	
____	____	____	4. Remove ordered medications from supply. Compare label on medication with the MAR or EMAR and check the five rights of medication administration. Scan bar code if using bar code medication administration (BCMA). If a discrepancy exists, recheck the client's chart and medication orders.	
____	____	____	5. Calculate correct drug dosage if necessary.	
____	____	____	6. Prepare selected medications.	
____	____	____	a. Unit dosage: Place packaged medications directly into medicine cup or lay them on tray without unwrapping them.	
____	____	____	b. Medications from a multidose bottle: Pour tablets or capsules into the container lid, and transfer them into medicine cup. Return any extra tablets to the bottle. Label all unlabeled medications. Break only scored tablets, if necessary, using a pill cutter to obtain proper dosage.	
____	____	____	c. Medications from a bingo card: Snap the bubble containing the correct medication directly over the medication cup. Do not touch the medication.	
____	____	____	d. Swallowing difficulty: If client has trouble swallowing tablets, grind with mortar and pestle or other drug-crushing device until smooth. Mix powder in small amount of pudding or applesauce. Do not crush enteric-coated tablets or extended-release tablets.	
____	____	____	e. Liquid medications: Remove cap and place on countertop with the inside up. Hold bottle so label is against palm of hand. Fill until bottom of meniscus (the surface of the fluid that appears curved) is at desired dosage. Discard excess poured liquid from cup into sink; do not pour it back into the bottle. Label medication.	

PROCEDURE 28-1
Administering Oral Medications (*Continued*)

Goal: To provide a safe, effective, economical route for administering medications; to provide sustained drug action with minimal discomfort.

Excellent	Satisfactory	Needs Practice		Comments
___	___	___	7. Take medications directly to client's room. Keep medications in sight at all times.	
___	___	___	8. Compare name on MAR with name on client's identification band using two separate identifiers (e.g., name, medical record number, Social Security number, or birth date). Do not administer medications if the client is not wearing an identification band. Scan client's identification bracelet if using bar code medication administration.	
___	___	___	9. Complete any preadministration assessment (e.g., blood pressure, pulse) required for the specific medication to be given.	
___	___	___	10. Compare medication to MAR, and recheck the five rights of medication administration. If using unit-dose medication, unwrap the medication and place it in the cup before checking the five rights of the next medication.	
___	___	___	11. Explain the medication's purpose to the client.	
___	___	___	12. Assist client to sitting position if necessary. Give the medication cup and glass of water to the client.	
___	___	___	13. If client cannot hold the medication cup, place it to the client's lips and introduce the medication into his or her mouth. If a tablet or capsule falls on the floor, discard and repeat preparation.	
___	___	___	14. Stay with client until he or she swallows all medications. Look inside client's mouth if the client is cognitively impaired or has difficulty swallowing.	
___	___	___	15. Dispose of soiled supplies, and wash hands.	
___	___	___	16. Record time at which medication was administered and any preadministration assessment data collected. Note the time that post-administration assessments to assess effectiveness are due for PRN medications. If a medication has been held, note this (usually by circling the medication) and give the reason the medication was not given.	

Procedure Checklists for Craven and Hirnle's Fundamentals of Nursing: Human Health and Function, 6th edition

Name _____ Date _____

Unit _____ Position _____

Instructor/Evaluator: _____ Position _____

PROCEDURE 28-2
Administering Medication by Metered-Dose Inhaler

Goal: To deliver a premeasured dose of medication to the bronchial airways and lungs.

Excellent	Satisfactory	Needs Practice		Comments
____	____	____	1. Check medication order and assess client allergies (see Procedure 28-1, Steps 1 to 5).	
____	____	____	2. Assist the client to sitting or standing position. Perform the second medication check of five rights.	
____	____	____	3. Instruct the client on assembly of medication canister, inhalation mouthpiece, and spacer device if needed. Instruct the client to attach the medication canister to the inhaler mouthpiece by inserting the metal stem into the long end of the mouthpiece. Teach client to shake the canister and spacer several times.	
____	____	____	4. Steps 4 through 6 need to occur smoothly, one right after the other. Ask client to breathe out through his or her mouth.	
____	____	____	5. Assist the client to position the mouthpiece 1 to 2 inches from his or her open mouth. If using a spacer, have client place spacer's mouthpiece into mouth, forming a secure seal. Instruct the client to breathe in slowly through the mouth. As the client starts inhaling, instruct the client to press the canister down to release one dose of the medication.	
____	____	____	6. Instruct the client to hold his or her breath for 10 seconds (if possible) and then to exhale slowly through pursed lips.	
____	____	____	7. Wait at least 1 minute before administration of a second puff by metered-dose inhaler (MDI).	
____	____	____	8. Wash hands and clean mouthpiece. If steroid medication was administered, have client rinse mouth.	
____	____	____	9. Reassess ease of breathing, respiratory rate, accessory muscle use, and breath sounds.	
____	____	____	10. Document medication administration and client status before and after administration.	

Modification for Using a Spacer With an MDI

____	____	____	11. Attach the spacer to the inhaler mouthpiece. Instruct the client to exhale and then place the mouthpiece in the mouth, closing his or her lips around the mouthpiece. Depress the medication canister and have the client inhale until the medication from the chamber is gone. Advise the client to take two or three short breaths to get all the medication from the spacer.	

Procedure Checklists for Craven and Hirnle's Fundamentals
of Nursing: Human Health and Function, 6th edition

Name _____ Date _____

Unit _____ Position _____

Instructor/Evaluator: _____ Position _____

Excellent	Satisfactory	Needs Practice	PROCEDURE 28-3 **Withdrawing Medication From a Vial**	
			Goal: To withdraw a precise amount of medication from a vial while maintaining asepsis.	**Comments**
___	___	___	1. Check medication order and compare the name of the ordered medication with the label on the medication vial. Complete Steps 1 through 5 in Procedure 28-1.	
___	___	___	2. Assemble needle and syringe.	
___	___	___	3. Pick up vial. If medication has been reconstituted or is in suspension, place the vial between your palms, rotating or rolling the vial back and forth. Do not shake the vial.	
___	___	___	4. Remove metal cap from vial, cleanse top of vial with alcohol wipe, and remove guard from needle. If multidose vial is being used (e.g., withdrawing insulin), date the vial when opened and discard on expiration date. Cleanse the vial top with alcohol prior to withdrawal.	
___	___	___	5. Pull back on barrel of syringe to draw in a volume of air equal to the volume of the ordered medication dose. Holding the vial between the thumb and fingers of the nondominant hand, insert needle through the rubber stopper into the air space— not the solution—in the vial and inject air.	
___	___	___	6. Invert the vial and withdraw the ordered dose of medication by pulling back on the plunger. Make sure that the needle is in the solution to be withdrawn.	
___	___	___	7. Expel air bubbles and adjust dose if necessary.	
___	___	___	8. Remove needle from vial and cover the needle with guard. Wash hands.	

Procedure Checklists for Craven and Hirnle's Fundamentals of Nursing: Human Health and Function, 6th edition

Name _____ Date _____

Unit _____ Position _____

Instructor/Evaluator: _____ Position _____

Excellent	Satisfactory	Needs Practice	PROCEDURE 28-4 **Withdrawing Medication From an Ampule**	Comments
			Goal: To withdraw the full dose of medication from an ampule safely while maintaining asepsis.	
____	____	____	1. Check medication order and make sure the solution in the ampule matches the ordered solution. Complete Steps 1 through 5 in Procedure 28-1.	
____	____	____	2. Assemble filter needle and syringe.	
____	____	____	3. Pick up ampule and flick its upper stem several times with a fingernail.	
____	____	____	4. Wrap a sterile gauze pad or alcohol wipe around the ampule's neck before breaking the neck along the scored line with an outward snapping motion. Always break away from your body.	
____	____	____	5. Discard the broken neck appropriately, and prepare to withdraw medication from the ampule using one of the following methods.	
____	____	____	a. Place the ampule upright on a flat surface, insert the needle in the solution, and withdraw the correct amount of medication by pulling up on the plunger. Do not touch the needle to the glass rim.	
____	____	____	b. Invert the ampule or tilt it sideways. Insert the needle into the solution; pull back on the plunger, and withdraw the proper dose of medication.	
____	____	____	6. Remove the needle from the solution. Hold the needle upright, inspect the syringe, and dispel any air that may have been drawn into the syringe. Make sure that the syringe contains the right amount of medication. Expel any extra medication into a container.	
____	____	____	7. Cover the filter needle with a safety guard and change the needle. Discard ampule in sharps container.	
____	____	____	8. Wash hands.	

Procedure Checklists for Craven and Hirnle's Fundamentals
of Nursing: Human Health and Function, 6th edition

Name _____ Date _____

Unit _____ Position _____

Instructor/Evaluator: _____ Position _____

Excellent	Satisfactory	Needs Practice	PROCEDURE 28-5 **Drawing Up Two Medications in a Syringe** **Goal:** To minimize the number of injections a client receives; to prevent contaminating one vial of medication with medication from the other vial.	Comments
____	____	____	1. Compare medications to the MAR. Complete Steps 1 through 5 of Procedure 28-1.	
____	____	____	2. Cleanse tops of both vials with antiseptic.	
____	____	____	3. With syringe, aspirate a volume of air equal to the medication dose from first medication (Vial A).	
____	____	____	4. Inject air into Vial A, being careful that the needle does not touch the solution.	
____	____	____	5. Remove syringe from Vial A.	
____	____	____	a. Aspirate volume of air equal to the medication dose from second medication (Vial B).	
____	____	____	b. Inject air into Vial B.	
____	____	____	6. Invert Vial B, and withdraw the required volume of medication into syringe. Expel all air bubbles, and withdraw needle from Vial B.	
____	____	____	7. Determine what the total combined volume of the two medications would measure on the syringe scale.	
____	____	____	8. Insert needle into Vial A, invert vial, and carefully withdraw required volume of medication (as in Step 6).	
____	____	____	9. Withdraw needle from Vial A and replace needle guard.	
____	____	____	10. Check medication and dosage before returning or discarding vials.	
			Modification for Insulin	
____	____	____	1. Wash hands.	
____	____	____	2. When preparing insulin in suspension, gently rotate vials between palms of hands to mix the suspension.	
____	____	____	3. Follow Steps 2 through 8 as above.	
____	____	____	4. Establish a routine order for drawing up insulin. The shorter-acting regular insulin is drawn up first, followed by the cloudy intermediate-acting insulin. Glargine (Lantus) insulin cannot be mixed with other types of insulin.	

Procedure Checklists for Craven and Hirnle's Fundamentals
of Nursing: Human Health and Function, 6th edition

Name _____   Date _____

Unit _____   Position _____

Instructor/Evaluator: _____   Position _____

Excellent	Satisfactory	Needs Practice	PROCEDURE 28-6 **Administering Intradermal Injections** **Goal:** To administer medication into the dermal tissue to screen for an allergic (antigen–antibody) dermal reaction, to screen for tuberculosis, or to administer local anesthesia.	Comments
____	____	____	1. Check medication order. See Procedure 28-1, Steps 1 through 5.	
____	____	____	2. Assemble needle and syringe.	
____	____	____	3. Remove needle guard and withdraw medication from vial (see Procedure 28-3).	
____	____	____	4. Identify client by two identifiers (name, medical record number, Social Security number, or birth date), checking identification bracelet. Scan bracelet if using bar code medication administration. Explain procedure to client. Repeat check of five rights.	
____	____	____	5. Don gloves. Select injection site that is relatively hairless and free from tenderness, swelling, scarring, and inflammation.	
____	____	____	6. Cleanse the site with an antimicrobial swab and then allow the skin to dry.	
____	____	____	7. Remove needle guard. Hold syringe in dominant hand. Gently pull skin distal to intended injection site taut with nondominant hand.	
____	____	____	8. Holding syringe from above, at 10- to 15-degree angle (almost parallel to skin), gently insert needle, bevel up, about an eighth of an inch until dermis barely covers bevel.	
____	____	____	9. Stabilize needle; inject medication slowly over 3 to 5 seconds while watching for a small wheal or blister to appear	
____	____	____	10. Withdraw needle at the same angle at which it was inserted. Do not wipe or massage site.	
____	____	____	11. Do not recap needle. Dispose of syringe and needle in sharps container.	
____	____	____	12. Record time and site of injection according to agency protocol.	
____	____	____	13. Instruct client when to return for reading of response—15 to 60 minutes after injection for allergy testing, and usually 48 to 72 hours after injection for tuberculin skin testing.	

Procedure Checklists for Craven and Hirnle's Fundamentals
of Nursing: Human Health and Function, 6th edition

Name _____ Date _____

Unit _____ Position _____

Instructor/Evaluator: _____ Position _____

PROCEDURE 28-7
Administering Subcutaneous Injections

Goal: To ensure more rapid absorption and action of a drug than can be achieved orally; to administer drugs to clients who are unable to take oral medications (e.g., unconscious, nausea/vomiting, NPO status); to administer medications that are not active by the oral route or are inactivated by digestive enzymes (e.g., heparin, insulin).

Excellent	Satisfactory	Needs Practice		Comments
____	____	____	1. Check medication order. See Procedure 28-1, Steps 1 through 5.	
____	____	____	2. Assemble needle and syringe.	
____	____	____	3. Remove needle guard and withdraw medication from container (see Procedures 28-3 and 28-4).	
____	____	____	4. Assess allergies. Identify client by two identifiers. Scan bracelet if using bar code medication administration. Explain procedure to client. Recheck five rights.	
____	____	____	5. Don gloves.	
____	____	____	6. Select an injection site that is free from tenderness, swelling, scarring, and inflammation.	
____	____	____	7. Cleanse site with antiseptic swab, using a circular motion from center toward outside. Allow area to dry thoroughly.	
____	____	____	8. Remove needle guard. Hold syringe in dominant hand. Place nondominant hand on either side of injection site. Spread or bunch skin to stabilize site and identify subcutaneous tissue.	
____	____	____	9. Hold syringe between thumb and forefinger of dominant hand (like a dart). Inject needle quickly at a 45- to 90-degree angle depending on the amount of subcutaneous tissue. Release bunched skin.	
____	____	____	10. Inject medication with slow, even pressure.	
____	____	____	11. Remove needle quickly at the same angle at which it was inserted while supporting the surrounding tissue with your nondominant hand. Apply gentle pressure to the site with a gauze square after the needle is withdrawn. Do not massage the site.	
____	____	____	12. Assist client to a position of comfort.	
____	____	____	13. Do not recap needle. Activate the needle guard. Dispose of syringe and needle in sharps container.	
____	____	____	14. Wash hands.	
____	____	____	15. Document according to agency protocol.	

Excellent	Satisfactory	Needs Practice	PROCEDURE 28-7 **Administering Subcutaneous Injections (*Continued*)**	Comments
			Goal: To ensure more rapid absorption and action of a drug than can be achieved orally; to administer drugs to clients who are unable to take oral medications (e.g., unconscious, nausea/vomiting, NPO status); to administer medications that are not active by the oral route or are inactivated by digestive enzymes (e.g., heparin, insulin).	

Modifications for Insulin Administration

- Routine aspiration is not necessary (ADA, 2003).
- Systematically rotate injection sites to prevent lipodystrophy and variable insulin absorption.
- Explain to the client that absorption differs depending on the site. The abdomen allows the fastest absorption, followed by arms, thighs, and buttocks (ADA, 2003). Exercise of a muscle group increases absorption.
- Instruct clients who self-administer insulin to always check the bottle label and draw up insulin in the same order each time.
- Insulin pens are increasingly used by diabetic clients for insulin administration. To use an insulin pen:
  1. Load cartridge with prescribed insulin.
  2. Screw on pen needle.
  3. Dial in desired dose.
  4. Inject needle into appropriate site and press button to deliver insulin.
  5. Remove and properly dispose of needle.
- For premixed insulins, prior to dosing, shake pen to mix insulins well.

Modifications for Heparin Administration

- The abdomen (avoiding the area 1 to 2 inches on either side of the umbilicus) is the most frequently used site because the lack of major muscle groups or muscle activity in the abdomen is thought to reduce the chance of hematoma formation.
- Roll or gently bunch the tissue between thumb and forefinger to ensure that heparin is administered into subcutaneous tissue. Do not tightly pinch the skin.
- Because heparin is an anticoagulant, do not aspirate for a blood return or massage the site after injection.
- After injection, slowly and smoothly withdraw the needle to prevent leakage into subcutaneous tissue.

Procedure Checklists for Craven and Hirnle's Fundamentals of Nursing: Human Health and Function, 6th edition

Name _____   Date _____

Unit _____   Position _____

Instructor/Evaluator: _____   Position _____

Excellent	Satisfactory	Needs Practice	PROCEDURE 28-8 **Administering Intramuscular Injections** **Goal:** To administer medication deeply into muscle tissue, without injury to the client; to administer a medication that requires absorption and onset of action quicker than the oral route without irritating the subcutaneous tissues.	Comments
____	____	____	1. Check medication order. See Procedure 28-1, Steps 1 through 5. Assemble needle and syringe.	
____	____	____	2. Prepare needle, syringe, and medication by following the appropriate steps in Procedures 28-3 or 28-4. If medication is known to be irritating to subcutaneous tissues, replace needle after withdrawing medication.	
____	____	____	3. Assess for allergies. Identify client by two identifiers. Scan bracelet if using bar code medication administration. Explain procedure to client. Recheck five rights.	
____	____	____	4. Don gloves. Assist client to a comfortable position, and expose only the area to be injected.	
____	____	____	5. Select appropriate injection site by inspecting muscle size and integrity. Consider volume of medication to be injected.	
____	____	____	6. Use anatomic landmarks to locate the exact injection site.	
____	____	____	7. Cleanse the site with antiseptic swab, wiping from center of site and rotating outward.	
____	____	____	8. Remove needle guard. Hold syringe between thumb and forefinger of dominant hand, like a dart. Spread skin at the site with nondominant hand. Encourage the client to relax the muscle or use distraction techniques.	
____	____	____	9. Insert needle quickly at a 90-degree angle to the client's skin surface.	
____	____	____	10. Stabilize syringe barrel by grasping with nondominant hand. a. Aspirate slowly by pulling back on plunger with dominant hand.	
____	____	____	b. If no blood appears, inject medication slowly.	
____	____	____	c. If blood appears in syringe, remove needle, dispose of syringe, and prepare new medication.	
____	____	____	11. Withdraw needle while pressing antiseptic swab above site.	
____	____	____	12. Apply gentle pressure at the site with dry gauze.	

PROCEDURE 28-8

Administering Intramuscular Injections (*Continued*)

Goal: To administer medication deeply into muscle tissue, without injury to the client; to administer a medication that requires absorption and onset of action quicker than the oral route without irritating the subcutaneous tissues.

Excellent	Satisfactory	Needs Practice		Comments

13. Do not recap needle. Activate needle guard. Dispose of equipment in sharps container.
14. Wash hands.
15. Record medication and client response according to agency protocol.

Variations for Z-Track Injection

- Manufacturers' guidelines for certain medications advise "for deep IM use only" or "given deeply into the body of a relatively large muscle." Z-track method is then the recommended technique.

1. When preparing the injection site, pull the skin and subcutaneous tissues about 1 to 1.5 inches to one side of the selected site.
2. Insert the syringe at a 90-degree angle. Do not release your nondominant hand that is stretching the skin to stabilize the syringe.
3. Aspirate and hold the syringe with one hand, and then administer medication while continuing traction on skin.
4. Leave needle inserted an additional 10 seconds.
5. Simultaneously remove needle along the line of insertion and release traction on skin.

Procedure Checklists for Craven and Hirnle's Fundamentals
of Nursing: Human Health and Function, 6th edition

Name _____   Date _____

Unit _____   Position _____

Instructor/Evaluator: _____   Position _____

Excellent	Satisfactory	Needs Practice	PROCEDURE 28-9 **Administering Medications By Intravenous Bolus (less than 5 minutes)** **Goal:** To achieve high blood levels of a medication in a short period; to achieve immediate and maximal effects of a medication.	Comments
____	____	____	1. Check medication order. See Procedure 28-1, Steps 1 through 5.	
____	____	____	2. If medication has not been prepared and labeled by pharmacy, the nurse prepares the medication. Draw up ordered medication from vial or ampule. Read package insert for proper amount and solution for dilution. Label syringe with name of medication and dose. Remove needle and dispose of it properly.	
____	____	____	3. Assess client allergies. Identify the client with two identifiers and recheck the five rights. Scan client's identification bracelet if using bar code medication administration.	
____	____	____	4. Explain procedure to the client.	
____	____	____	5. Assess IV site for signs of infiltration or phlebitis.	
____	____	____	6. Don clean gloves.	
			Administering Medication into an Existing IV Line	
____	____	____	1. Select injection port or "Y" site in IV tubing closest to the IV insertion site. Clean port with antimicrobial swab.	
____	____	____	2. Uncap the syringe. Steady the port with your nondominant hand while inserting the syringe or needleless device into center of injection port.	
____	____	____	3. Occlude the tubing by folding it between your fingers.	
____	____	____	4. Pull back on plunger to assess for blood return.	
____	____	____	5. Inject the medication slowly into the IV port at the prescribed rate. It is helpful to use a watch to time the administration rate.	
____	____	____	6. If IV medication and IV solution in tubing are incompatible, flush line with normal saline solution while occluding catheter above port. Administer medication at prescribed rate; reflush with 10 mL of sterile normal saline solution and release occlusion.	

PROCEDURE 28-9
Administering Medications By Intravenous Bolus (less than 5 minutes) (*Continued*)

Excellent	Satisfactory	Needs Practice	**Goal:** To achieve high blood levels of a medication in a short period; to achieve immediate and maximal effects of a medication.	Comments
			Administering the Drug into an Intermittent Infusion Device or Lock Device	
____	____	____	1. Don gloves. Clean port with antimicrobial swab using friction.	
____	____	____	2. Stabilize port with your nondominant hand and insert syringe with 1 mL normal saline solution into injection port.	
____	____	____	3. Release the clamp on the extension tubing of the medication lock. Aspirate gently and check for blood return.	
____	____	____	4. Gently flush with normal saline by pushing slowly on the syringe plunger. Observe the insertion site while inserting the saline. Remove the syringe.	
____	____	____	5. Insert syringe with medication into injection port. Inject medication slowly at the prescribed rate. Use watch to time administration rate. Remove syringe. Do not force the injection if resistance is felt. Remove medication syringe from port.	
____	____	____	6. Insert syringe with 1 to 3 mL of normal saline into injection port and gently flush the port with saline. To gain positive pressure, clamp the IV tubing as you are still flushing the last of the saline into the medication lock. Remove the syringe from the injection port.	
____	____	____	7. Dispose of used syringes properly, remove gloves, and wash hands.	
____	____	____	8. Document medication administration.	
____	____	____	9. Evaluate and chart the client's response to medication therapy and document according to agency policy.	

Procedure Checklists for Craven and Hirnle's Fundamentals
of Nursing: Human Health and Function, 6th edition

Name _____   Date _____

Unit _____   Position _____

Instructor/Evaluator: _____   Position _____

Excellent	Satisfactory	Needs Practice	PROCEDURE 28-10 **Administering Intravenous Medications Using Intermittent Infusion Technique**	Comments
			Goal: To maintain therapeutic levels of medication in client's blood; to dilute irritating intravenous (IV) medications; to prevent complications associated with bolus administration by delivering medications over a longer period; to prevent combining incompatible medications.	
			Administering IV Medications When Using Syringe Pump and Heparin Lock	
____	____	____	1. Check medication order. See Procedure 28-1, Steps 1 through 5.	
____	____	____	2. Prepare the medication syringe and IV tubing. Examine the syringe for any air bubbles and expel any that are present. Attach the syringe to the extension tubing, and gently push the syringe plunger to prime the tubing. Cover adaptor.	
____	____	____	3. Secure the medication syringe into the pump with the flange of the syringe in the clamp's groove.	
____	____	____	4. Assess for client allergies. Confirm the client's identity by checking two identifiers. Scan the patient's bracelet if using bar code medication administration. Recheck the five rights and explain the procedure to the client.	
____	____	____	5. Assess the IV site for inflammation or infiltration.	
____	____	____	6. Don gloves.	
____	____	____	7. Attach syringe with normal saline into the lock device. Flush lock with normal saline.	
____	____	____	8. Attach tubing to lock device. Secure IV tubing to IV site with tape.	
____	____	____	9. Program the pump for the appropriate infusion speed and press the start key. The medication syringe label often indicates the suggested infusion speed, typically 30 to 60 minutes. If uncertain, consult a drug reference handbook or pharmacist.	
____	____	____	10. Document medication administration.	
____	____	____	11. Assess the client and infusion device 5 to 10 minutes after infusion has begun.	
____	____	____	12. When the completion alarm sounds, return to client's room and press the pump's stop key.	
____	____	____	13. Don gloves. Remove tubing from lock device. Attach syringe with 1 to 3 mL normal saline or heparin flush solution and flush lock.	

PROCEDURE 28-10
Administering Intravenous Medications Using Intermittent Infusion Technique (*Continued*)

Excellent	Satisfactory	Needs Practice		Comments

Goal: To maintain therapeutic levels of medication in client's blood; to dilute irritating intravenous (IV) medications; to prevent complications associated with bolus administration by delivering medications over a longer period; to prevent combining incompatible medications.

___ ___ ___   14. Replace lock with new sterile cap.
___ ___ ___   15. Dispose of syringes in proper container. Wash hands.

Administering Intermittent IV Medication into Primary IV Line Using an Electronic Infusion Device (EID)

___ ___ ___   1. Check medication order. See Procedure 28-1, Steps 1 through 5. Prepare medication, tubing, and EID according to procedures described earlier.
___ ___ ___   2. Assess client allergies. Confirm client's identity using two identifiers and check five rights again.
___ ___ ___   3. Assess the IV site for inflammation or infiltration.
___ ___ ___   4. Position infusion bags so that the medication (secondary) bag is at or above the level of the primary IV solution. Insert secondary line into the adaptor port.
___ ___ ___   5. Check compatibility of medications to be administered with the IV solution being infused and any other infusing medications. If medication is not compatible with primary IV solution, clamp primary IV tubing above injection port, attach syringe with 20-mL of normal saline flush solution, and flush IV line. Do not administer IV medication through tubing that is infusing blood products or total parenteral nutrition.
___ ___ ___   6. Clean the access port on the primary IV infusion tubing using an antimicrobial swab.
___ ___ ___   7. Connect secondary (piggyback) line to injection port or "Y" site on IV tubing closest to IV insertion site.
___ ___ ___   8. Program the EID with the correct volume and infusion rate for secondary infusion. Release clamps and press start button.
___ ___ ___   9. When medication has infused, discard medication bag and tubing (or reserve for next medication infusion) according to agency guidelines.
___ ___ ___   10. Wash hands.
___ ___ ___   11. Document medication administration and add IV volume to IV intake.

Name _____   Date _____

Unit _____   Position _____

Instructor/Evaluator: _____   Position _____

Excellent	Satisfactory	Needs Practice	PROCEDURE 29-1 **Initiating Intravenous Therapy** **Goal:** To maintain or replace fluids for daily body fluid requirements; to provide electrolytes to maintain or restore electrolyte balance; to deliver glucose and nutrients for use as an energy source; to deliver medication or blood products.	Comments
____	____	____	1. Verify the order for IV therapy with the physician's order, including solution type, amount, additives, and infusion.	
____	____	____	2. Gather all equipment and bring it to the client's bedside.	
____	____	____	3. Identify the client using two separate identifiers.	
____	____	____	4. Explain the rationale for IV therapy and the procedure.	
____	____	____	5. Perform hand hygiene.	
			Preparing the Solution	
____	____	____	6. Remove the IV solution bag from the outer plastic covering (if not already done). Open all other equipment packages, maintaining sterility of the equipment.	
____	____	____	7. Grasp the IV administration set and close the flow clamp on the tubing. Attach an extension set tubing to the administration set if necessary.	
____	____	____	8. Remove the protective cap or tear the tab from the tubing insertion port on the solution container; remove the protective covering from the spike on the administration tubing. Hold the port carefully and firmly with one hand, then quickly insert the spike into the port with the other hand.	
____	____	____	9. Invert the solution container and hang it on the IV pole with the infusion pump. Compress the drip chamber until it is approximately half full. Remove the protective cap from the end of the infusion tubing (or extension set, if used) if necessary; direct the end of the tubing toward a receptacle. Open the flow clamp on the tubing and allow the fluid to run through the tubing until all the air has been removed and the entire length of the tubing is filled with solution; then close the flow clamp.	
____	____	____	10. Attach the solution and tubing to the infusion control device according to the manufacturer's instructions. Apply label to the solution container if one has not already been applied by the pharmacy.	

PROCEDURE 29-1

Initiating Intravenous Therapy (*Continued*)

Excellent	Satisfactory	Needs Practice	**Goal:** To maintain or replace fluids for daily body fluid requirements; to provide electrolytes to maintain or restore electrolyte balance; to deliver glucose and nutrients for use as an energy source; to deliver medication or blood products.	Comments

Selecting the Insertion Site

_____ _____ _____   11. Place the client in a comfortable, reclining position, leaving the arm in a dependent position. Place a towel or protective pad under the extremity to be used. Inspect and palpate the client's extremity to identify an appropriate vein. Select the puncture site. If long-term therapy is anticipated, start with a vein at the most distal site so that you can move proximally as needed for subsequent IV insertion sites.

_____ _____ _____   12. Put on clean gloves and apply a tourniquet about 6 inches (15 cm) above the intended puncture site. Ensure that the ends of the tourniquet are positioned away from the intended insertion site. Check for a radial pulse. If it isn't present, release the tourniquet and reapply it with less tension.

_____ _____ _____   13. Lightly palpate the vein with the index and middle fingers of your nondominant hand. Stretch the skin to anchor the vein. If the vein feels hard or ropelike, select another site.

Inserting the Device and Initiating Therapy

_____ _____ _____   14. Administer a local anesthetic if ordered. If a topical anesthetic is ordered, ensure adequate time from the application of the topical agent to insertion.

_____ _____ _____   15. Clean the site using the approved antimicrobial agent according to facility policy. Work in a circular motion outward from the site to a diameter of 2 to 4 inches (5 to 10 cm), and allow the agent to dry. If facility policy permits, clip the area around the intended insertion site for a distance of up to 2 inches if the site is hairy.

_____ _____ _____   16. Grasp the device. Using the thumb of your nondominant hand, stretch the skin taut below the puncture site. If using a vein in the hand, position the hand in a slightly flexed position to keep the skin taut. Tell the client that you are about to insert the device and that you need him or her to remain still.

_____ _____ _____   17. Hold the needle bevel up at an angle of approximately 10 to 15 degrees and enter the skin parallel to the vein. Insert the device directly through the skin and into the vein in one motion either from

PROCEDURE 29-1
Initiating Intravenous Therapy (*Continued*)

Excellent	Satisfactory	Needs Practice	**Goal:** To maintain or replace fluids for daily body fluid requirements; to provide electrolytes to maintain or restore electrolyte balance; to deliver glucose and nutrients for use as an energy source; to deliver medication or blood products.	**Comments**
			directly over the vein or from the side. You will feel a sense of release or a pop as you enter the vein. Check for blood return and then advance the device, maintaining the device parallel to the skin until the hub is at the insertion site.	
____	____	____	18. Remove the tourniquet quickly. While holding the hub with your nondominant hand, attach the end of the infusion tubing to the device.	
			Applying a Dressing	
____	____	____	19. Apply a dressing (most commonly a transparent, semipermeable dressing) to the site. Alternatively, secure the device with nonallergenic tape and cover with a 2 × 2 gauze.	
____	____	____	20. Loop any IV tubing on the client's extremity and secure with tape.	
____	____	____	21. Label the dressing with the date and time of insertion, device type, gauge, and size and your initials.	
____	____	____	22. Begin the infusion, setting the infusion pump to the prescribed rate of flow. Assess the flow of the solution and infusion control device function. Inspect the site for signs of infiltration.	
			Providing Ongoing Care	
____	____	____	23. Dispose of all equipment and remove gloves. Perform hand hygiene.	
____	____	____	24. Apply an armboard or site protection device and secure as necessary.	
____	____	____	25. Assist the client to a comfortable position. Assess the client's tolerance of the procedure.	
____	____	____	26. Document the procedure, including the date and time of the venipuncture, device type, gauge, and length, location of insertion site and appearance, type and flow rate of the IV solution, client's response (including adverse reactions), client teaching performed, and client's understanding of the teaching.	
____	____	____	27. Monitor infusion rate, condition of IV site, and client complaints, initially approximately 30 minutes after beginning the infusion and then according to facility policy. Change dressing, tubing, and solutions according to facility policy.	

Procedure Checklists for Craven and Hirnle's Fundamentals of Nursing: Human Health and Function, 6th edition

Name _____ Date _____

Unit _____ Position _____

Instructor/Evaluator: _____ Position _____

Excellent	Satisfactory	Needs Practice	PROCEDURE 29-2 **Monitoring an Intravenous Infusion**	Comments
			Goal: To provide a safe, patent route for infusion of IV therapy; to ensure correct infusion of IV fluids; to detect IV complications promptly.	
___	___	___	1. Identify client with two separate identifiers. Compare IV fluid currently infusing with the ordered solution.	
___	___	___	2. Inspect the rate of flow at least every hour. For gravity-regulated IVs, check actual flow rate for 15 seconds and multiply by 4 for the minute rate. Compare the assessed rate with prescribed flow rate. If the infusion is ahead of schedule, slow it so the infusion will complete at the planned time. If infusion is behind schedule, review hospital policy before increasing flow rate; some agencies require a physician's order to increase the rate of flow. If EID is used, the hourly infusion rate in mL/hr is programmed into the machine. Most EID manufacturers require use of cassette tubing unique to their machines.	
___	___	___	3. Inspect the system for leakage; if present, locate the source. Tighten all connections within the system. If leak persists, slow IV flow rate to keep vein open and replace tubing with sterile set.	
___	___	___	4. Inspect the tubing for kinks or blockages. Loosely coil tubing and place it on the bed.	
___	___	___	5. Inspect the insertion site and dressing for leakage of IV solution.	
___	___	___	6. Inspect the infusion site for infiltration. Infiltration occurs when the needle becomes dislodged from the vein and IV fluid flows into the interstitial tissue. Look for signs of infiltration, including decreased flow rate, swelling, pallor, coolness, and discomfort at or above needle insertion site. If signs are present, change the IV site. If a large amount of fluid has infiltrated, elevate the arm above the heart on several pillows.	
___	___	___	7. Inspect arm above the insertion point for signs of phlebitis, including redness, swelling, warmth, and pain along the vein above IV insertion site. If present, discontinue the IV and restart in another area. Ask the client to report burning or pain at the	

PROCEDURE 29-2
Monitoring an Intravenous Infusion (*Continued*)

Excellent	Satisfactory	Needs Practice	**Goal:** To provide a safe, patent route for infusion of IV therapy; to ensure correct infusion of IV fluids; to detect IV complications promptly.	Comments
			IV site. If you suspect phlebitis is present, notify the physician and check agency policy for treating phlebitis.	
___	___	___	8. Inspect the insertion site for bleeding.	
			9. Inspect the site for local manifestations, including redness, pus, warmth, induration, and pain, which may indicate that infection is present at the site. Inspect the client for systemic manifestations, including chills, fever, tachycardia, and hypotension, that may accompany local infection. Inspect the site for additional complications of IV therapy (e.g., fluid overload).	
___	___	___	10. Check EID alarm settings. Attend to all alarms in a timely manner.	
___	___	___	11. Although monitoring IV therapy is a nursing responsibility, if the client is able to comply, teach him or her to contact the nurse if the following occur:	
___	___	___	a. The flow rate changes suddenly.	
___	___	___	b. The fluid container is almost empty.	
___	___	___	c. Blood is in the tubing.	
___	___	___	d. The site becomes uncomfortable.	
			12. Chart any findings indicating complications of IV therapy (e.g., infiltration).	

Procedure Checklists for Craven and Hirnle's Fundamentals of Nursing: Human Health and Function, 6th edition

Name _____   Date _____

Unit _____   Position _____

Instructor/Evaluator: _____   Position _____

PROCEDURE 29-3
Peripheral IV Site Care

Goal: To protect the IV site from infection; to permit visual inspection of the IV site to promptly detect complications of therapy.

Excellent	Satisfactory	Needs Practice		Comments
____	____	____	1. Perform hand hygiene. Put on clean gloves. Place waterproof pad under IV site.	
____	____	____	2. Inspect site for signs of infection, infiltration, and thrombophlebitis.	
____	____	____	3. Hold catheter in place with your nondominant hand and gently remove dressing and tape. For transparent dressing, gently stretch the film horizontal to the skin.	
____	____	____	4. Clean the entry site with a chlorhexidine solution, using a circular motion and moving from the center outward. Allow the area to dry completely; do not blow or blot dry.	
____	____	____	5. Apply transparent semipermeable dressing to the IV site. Take care not to tape over the IV connection or IV tubing.	
____	____	____	6. Label dressing with date, time, and initials. Secure IV tubing with additional tape if necessary.	
____	____	____	7. Assess IV flow is accurate and system is patent.	
____	____	____	8. Remove gloves and perform hand hygiene. Document dressing change and observations.	

*Procedure Checklists for Craven and Hirnle's Fundamentals
of Nursing: Human Health and Function,* 6th edition

Name _____ Date _____

Unit _____ Position _____

Instructor/Evaluator: _____ Position _____

PROCEDURE 29-4
Central Venous Access Device (PICC) Site Care

Goal: To protect the IV site from infection; to permit visual inspection of the IV site to promptly detect complications of therapy.

Excellent	Satisfactory	Needs Practice		Comments
___	___	___	1. Perform hand hygiene. Place client in a comfortable position and explain procedure.	
___	___	___	2. Apply mask. Have client put on mask and turn head away from site. Prepare sterile field and place sterile drape around site.	
___	___	___	3. Assess insertion site for infection and phlebitis.	
___	___	___	4. Put on clean gloves. Stabilize catheter with thumb. Remove old dressing, stretching horizontally and then working proximally. Remove old gloves.	
___	___	___	5. Don sterile gloves and clean the area around the site with a chlorhexidine solution. Move in a circular fashion, cleaning from the insertion site outward 2 to 3 inches. Allow to dry; do not blow or blot.	
___	___	___	6. Re-dress the site with a transparent semipermeable dressing, according to agency policy. Secure tubing and all Luer lock connections.	
___	___	___	7. Label the dressing with date, time, and initials.	
___	___	___	8. Clamp all lines of device and remove injection caps. Cleanse catheter ends with antimicrobial swab and reapply new injection caps.	
___	___	___	9. Flush the catheter according to agency policy. Flush with 3 to 5 mL of NSS using a 10-mL syringe and 3 mL of heparin (100 U/mL). Use the "pulse-pause" technique, always ending with positive pressure by clamping prior to ending the flush.	
___	___	___	10. Discard all used items properly. Reposition the patient comfortably. Document dressing change and observations.	

Procedure Checklists for Craven and Hirnle's Fundamentals of Nursing: Human Health and Function, 6th edition

Name _____   Date _____

Unit _____   Position _____

Instructor/Evaluator: _____   Position _____

Excellent	Satisfactory	Needs Practice	PROCEDURE 29-5 **Changing Intravenous Solution and Tubing**	Comments
			Goal: To deliver IV therapy as ordered; to decrease risk of client infection.	
			Changing Solution Container	
___	___	___	1. Wash hands. Explain procedure to client.	
___	___	___	2. Compare solution with physician's order. Assess client allergies. Adhere to five rights of medication administration, including identifying the client with two separate identifiers.	
___	___	___	3. Remove IV bag from outer wrapper. Look for leaks or impurities in the bag and check the IV fluid bag for expiration date.	
___	___	___	4. Label solution container with client's name, solution type, additives, date, and time hung. If not already done, check prelabeled container with physician's order. Line up time strip with volume amount on bag or bottle. Record solution change in the client's record.	
___	___	___	5. Prepare container for spiking: a. If solution is in a plastic bag, remove plastic cover from entry nipple. Maintain sterility of nipple end.	
___	___	___	b. If solution is in a bottle, remove metal cap, metal disk, and rubber disk. Maintain sterility of bottle top.	
___	___	___	6. Close the clamp on the existing tubing. If using an electronic device, turn the device to the "hold" position.	
___	___	___	7. Take old solution container from pole and invert it. Quickly remove spike from used container, maintaining its sterility.	
___	___	___	8. Spike new IV container with firm push/twist motion and hang new container on IV pole. Alternatively, you can hang the IV bag, then spike the new container.	
___	___	___	9. Inspect tubing for air bubbles, and assess that drip chamber is half-full of solution.	
___	___	___	10. Reopen and adjust clamp to regulate flow rate or program EID, according to orders.	

PROCEDURE 29-5
Changing Intravenous Solution and Tubing (*Continued*)

Goal: To deliver IV therapy as ordered; to decrease risk of client infection.

Comments

Excellent	Satisfactory	Needs Practice	

Changing Solution and Tubing with Extension Tubing in Place

1. Follow Steps 1 to 4 of "Changing Solution Container."
2. Open new tubing package. Keep protective covers on spike.
3. Adjust roller clamp on new tubing to fully closed position.
4. Prepare new solution container as directed in Step 5 of "Changing Solution Container."
5. Maintaining sterility, remove protective cover from spike and insert spike into new solution container. Hang container and "prime" drip chamber by squeezing gently, allowing to fill half-full.
6. Remove protective cap from end of IV tubing, and adjust roller clamp to flush tubing with fluid. Replace protective cap.
7. If an electronic device is to be used, follow manufacturer's instructions for inserting tubing and setting infusion rate.
8. Adjust roller clamp on old tubing to close fully. Also, close the clamp on the short extension tubing connected to the IV catheter in the client's arm.
9. Remove the current infusion tubing from the resealable cap on the short extension IV tubing.
10. Using an antimicrobial swab, cleanse the resealable cap and insert the new IV tubing into the cap.
11. Open the clamp on the IV tubing and on the short extension tubing.
12. Program the EID or adjust roller clamp to start solution flowing according to physician's order.
13. Secure tubing with tape.
14. If dressing was removed, apply new dressing to IV site according to agency policy.
15. Label new tubing with date, time, and your initials. Label solution container with client's name, solution type, additives, date and time hung. Time label on IV container (if not already done). Record solution and tubing change.
16. Discard used equipment properly and perform hand hygiene.

Excellent	Satisfactory	Needs Practice	PROCEDURE 29-5 **Changing Intravenous Solution and Tubing (*Continued*)**	
			Goal: To deliver IV therapy as ordered; to decrease risk of client infection.	**Comments**
			Changing IV Tubing Connected Directly into the Hub of the IV Access Catheter	
——	——	——	1. Follow first four steps of "Changing Solution Container."	
——	——	——	2. Open new tubing package. Keep protective covers on spike and catheter adapter.	
——	——	——	3. Adjust roller clamp on new tubing to fully closed position.	
——	——	——	4. Prepare new solution container as directed in Step 5 of "Changing Solution Container."	
——	——	——	5. Maintaining sterility, remove protective cover from spike and insert spike into new solution container.	
——	——	——	6. Hang container and "prime" drip chamber by squeezing gently, allowing to fill half-full.	
——	——	——	7. Remove protective cap from end of IV tubing, and adjust roller clamp to flush tubing with fluid. Replace protective cap.	
——	——	——	8. Adjust roller clamp on old tubing to close fully.	
——	——	——	9. Place towel or disposable pad under extremity. Don clean, disposable gloves.	
——	——	——	10. Hold catheter hub with fingers of one hand (may use hemostat). With other hand, loosen old tubing using gentle twisting motion. *Note:* The dressing may have to be removed.	
——	——	——	11. Grasp new tubing, remove protective catheter cap, disconnect IV tubing, and Luer lock new tubing tightly into needle hub while continuing to stabilize catheter hub with other hand.	
——	——	——	12. Program the EID or adjust roller clamp to start solution flowing according to physician's order.	
——	——	——	13. Discard gloves.	
——	——	——	14. Secure tubing with tape.	
——	——	——	15. If dressing was removed, apply new dressing to IV site according to agency policy.	
——	——	——	16. Label new tubing with date, time, and your initials.	
——	——	——	17. Label solution container with client's name, solution type, additives, and date and time hung (if not already done). Record solution and tubing change.	

Procedure Checklists for Craven and Hirnle's Fundamentals of Nursing: Human Health and Function, 6th edition

Name _____   Date _____

Unit _____   Position _____

Instructor/Evaluator: _____   Position _____

Excellent	Satisfactory	Needs Practice		Comments
			PROCEDURE 29-6 # Converting to an Intermittent Infusion Device and Flushing **Goal:** To maintain patency of intermittently used IV access for IV medication and emergency IV access; to permit client increased mobility and freedom if continuous IV infusion is not required.	
			Beginning the Procedure	
___	___	___	1. Wash hands.	
___	___	___	2. Identify the client using two separate identifiers. Explain procedure to client.	
___	___	___	3. Assess IV site for signs of phlebitis, infiltration, or infection. If complications are detected, discontinue the IV and restart it in another site.	
___	___	___	4. Prepare syringe with heparin flush solution or saline solution according to agency policy and manufacturer's recommendations for the type of device in place (may use between 0.5 and 1 mL [peripheral], 2.5 and 3 mL [central line] heparin flush, or 1 and 3 mL normal saline). Label syringes.	
			Converting to IID when Extension Tubing is in Place	
___	___	___	1. Clamp off primary IV tubing	
___	___	___	2. Put on clean gloves. Clamp the extension tubing. Disconnect IV tubing from extension tubing.	
___	___	___	3. Cleanse port on extension tubing with antiseptic swab.	
___	___	___	4. Unclamp the extension set and insert a normal saline or heparin flush syringe into the cap. Flush with heparin or normal saline according to agency policy. Inject the recommended amount of saline or heparin flush, using pulsating technique, ending with 0.5 mL of solution remaining in syringe. Do not force if resistance is met. Reclamp the extension tubing and remove the syringe. Attach sterile end protector. *Note:* This procedure must be done at least every 8 hours or after each use of the catheter for IV medications to ensure catheter patency. Most agencies recommend changing IV locks every 72 hours to ensure patency and to prevent common complications of IV therapy.	

Excellent	Satisfactory	Needs Practice		Comments

PROCEDURE 29-6
Converting to an Intermittent Infusion Device and Flushing (*Continued*)

Goal: To maintain patency of intermittently used IV access for IV medication and emergency IV access; to permit client increased mobility and freedom if continuous IV infusion is not required.

——— ——— ———   5. Dispose of syringes in proper container. Remove gloves and dispose of them properly.

——— ——— ———   6. Tape adapter device and extension tubing.

——— ——— ———   7. Wash hands.

——— ——— ———   8. Document date, time, route, amount, and type of flush solution. Also document assessment of site.

Converting to IID with Extension Tubing when Extension Tubing Is Not Already in Place

——— ——— ———   1. If extension tubing is not in place, obtain the appropriate IID (saline lock) with extension tubing. Don clean gloves.

——— ——— ———   2. Clamp tubing of IV infusion with roller clamp.

——— ——— ———   3. Take extension tubing with IID out of package, keeping tip sterile. Hold in dominant hand between thumb and finger. Insert needleless syringe into port of extension tubing to prepare for flushing of the IV catheter.

——— ——— ———   4. Stabilize IV catheter hub firmly with nondominant hand as you disconnect IV tubing from the IV catheter with dominant hand. Quickly insert extension tubing with IID into IV catheter, twisting to the right to tighten.

——— ——— ———   5. Flush with heparin or normal saline according to agency policy. Inject the recommended amount of saline or heparin flush, using pulsating technique, ending with 0.5 mL of solution remaining in syringe. Do not force if resistance is met. Clamp the extension tubing. *Note:* This procedure must be done at least every 8 hours or after each use of the catheter for IV medications to ensure catheter patency. Most agencies recommend changing IV locks every 72 hours to ensure patency and to prevent common complications of IV therapy (e.g., phlebitis).

——— ——— ———   6. Dispose of syringes in proper container.

——— ——— ———   7. Tape IID with extension tubing to stabilize. Re-dress using transparent dressing if necessary.

——— ——— ———   8. Wash hands.

——— ——— ———   9. Document date, time, route, amount, and type of flush solution. Also document assessment of site.

PROCEDURE 29-6
Converting to an Intermittent Infusion Device and Flushing (*Continued*)

Goal: To maintain patency of intermittently used IV access for IV medication and emergency IV access; to permits client increased mobility and freedom if continuous IV infusion is not required.

Excellent	Satisfactory	Needs Practice		Comments

Converting to IID when No Extension Tubing Is Used

1. If extension tubing is not in place, obtain the appropriate IID (saline lock). Don clean gloves.
2. Clamp tubing of IV infusion with roller clamp.
3. Hold the catheter hub firmly with your non-dominant hand (a hemostat may be used if necessary). With dominant hand, quickly twist IV tubing to the left to loosen but not disconnect from IV catheter.
4. Take IID out of package, keeping tip sterile. Hold in dominant hand between thumb and finger.
5. Stabilize IV catheter with nondominant hand as you disconnect IV tubing. Quickly insert IID into IV catheter, twisting to the right to tighten.
6. Tape IID to stabilize. Redress using transparent dressing if necessary.
7. Swab injection port with antiseptic swab and allow to dry.
8. Insert the needleless syringe into the port and aspirate gently for evidence of blood return.
9. Inject the recommended amount of saline or heparin flush, using pulsating technique, ending with 0.5 mL of solution remaining in syringe. Do not force if resistance is met. *Note:* This procedure must be done at least every 8 hours or after each use of the catheter for IV medications to ensure catheter patency. Most agencies recommend changing IV locks every 72 hours to ensure patency and to prevent commonly associated complications of IV therapy (e.g., phlebitis).
10. Dispose of syringes in proper container.
11. Wash hands.
12. Document date, time, route, amount, and type of flush solution. Also document assessment of site.

Procedure Checklists for Craven and Hirnle's Fundamentals
of Nursing: Human Health and Function, 6th edition

Name _____ Date _____

Unit _____ Position _____

Instructor/Evaluator: _____ Position _____

			PROCEDURE 29-7	
			Administering Total Parenteral Nutrition	

Goal: To provide parenteral nutritional support to malnourished clients; to provide parenteral nutritional support to clients who are NPO for extended periods of time; to provide parenteral nutritional support to clients requiring bypass of the gastrointestinal tract for prolonged periods; to provide parenteral nutritional support to clients who have excessive metabolic needs due to trauma, cancer, or hypermetabolic states.

Excellent	Satisfactory	Needs Practice		Comments
			Monitoring TPN Therapy	
____	____	____	1. Schedule and assist client with chest x-ray after central catheter insertion.	
____	____	____	2. Confirm correct solution against physician's order. Check solution's expiration date. Assess client allergies. Identify the client with two separate identifiers and complete the five rights of medication administration. Set the EID for the proper infusion rate. *Note:* Solutions with more than 10% dextrose must be infused directly into a central catheter to rapidly dilute the solution and prevent thrombophlebitis. Constant flow rate helps prevent hyperglycemia and electrolyte imbalances.	
____	____	____	3. Inspect tubing and catheter connection for leaks or kinks. Tape all connections. Change tubing every 24 hours according to agency policy.	
____	____	____	4. Inspect insertion site for infiltration, thrombophlebitis, or drainage. If present, notify physician. The physician may order removal of the catheter and culture of the catheter tip.	
____	____	____	5. Monitor vital signs, including temperature, every 4 hours.	
____	____	____	6. Use the TPN line only for administration of TPN and lipids. Do not use the line for any other reason.	
____	____	____	7. Perform test for glucose as ordered (usually every 12 or 24 hours). Notify physician if abnormal.	
____	____	____	8. Monitor laboratory tests of electrolytes, BUN, glucose, as ordered, and report abnormal findings.	
____	____	____	9. Maintain accurate record of intake and output to monitor fluid balance.	
____	____	____	10. Weigh client daily and record.	
____	____	____	11. Inspect dressing once a shift for drainage and intactness. Change dressing whenever loose	

PROCEDURE 29-7
Administering Total Parenteral Nutrition (*Continued*)

Goal: To provide parenteral nutritional support to malnour-ished clients; to provide parenteral nutritional support to clients who are NPO for extended periods of time; to pro-vide parenteral nutritional support to clients requiring bypass of the gastrointestinal tract for prolonged periods; to provide parenteral nutritional support to clients who have excessive metabolic needs due to trauma, cancer, or hypermetabolic states.

Excellent	Satisfactory	Needs Practice		Comments

or moist, and perform site care at least every 48 hours.

Administering Intralipids

1. Check solution against physician's order. Inspect solution for separation of emulsion into layers or for froth. Do not use if present.
2. Wash your hands and don gloves.
3. Attach fat emulsion tubing to bottle. Prime tubing as for a conventional IV.
4. Identify client using two separate identifiers. Adhere to the five rights of medication administration. Assess client allergies.
5. Identify Y-port on tubing (below in-line filter).
6. Cleanse Y-port with antiseptic swab. Allow to dry. Insert connector into port. Secure with tape.
   Note: Lipids can be infused into a peripheral IV.
7. Adjust flow rate to infuse at 1.0 mL/min for adults and 0.1 mL/min for children. Infuse at this rate for 30 minutes while monitoring the client and vital signs every 10 minutes. If any adverse reactions occur, stop infusion and notify physician.
8. If no adverse reactions occur, adjust flow rate:
   a. Adults: 500 mL intralipid over 4 to 6 hours
   b. Children: up to 1 g/kg over 4 hours

Procedure Checklists for Craven and Hirnle's Fundamentals of Nursing: Human Health and Function, 6th edition

Name _____ Date _____

Unit _____ Position _____

Instructor/Evaluator: _____ Position _____

Excellent	Satisfactory	Needs Practice	PROCEDURE 29-8 **Administering a Blood Transfusion** **Goal:** To replace blood volume or blood components lost through trauma, surgery, or a disease process; to prevent complications from transfusing incompatible blood products.	Comments
____	____	____	1. Explain procedure to client. Have client sign consent form if required by hospital policy. Teach client what to report in the event of an adverse reaction, such as chills, back pain, headache, nausea or vomiting, rapid heart rate, rapid breathing, or skin rash.	
____	____	____	2. Administer any potentially ordered premedications, such as diphenhydramine (Benadryl).	
____	____	____	3. Obtain client's vital signs, including temperature.	
____	____	____	4. With another RN, a physician, or other licensed staff member at the client's bedside, verify the blood component and the client's identity by comparing the laboratory blood record with:	
____	____	____	a. The client's name and identification number, both verbally and against client's identification band	
____	____	____	b. The blood unit number on the blood bag label	
____	____	____	c. The blood group and Rh factor on the blood bag label Also verify the kind of blood component and the expiration date on the blood label. Document verification by both RN signatures on transfusion record.	
____	____	____	5. Wash your hands. Put on clean gloves.	
____	____	____	6. Open Y-type blood administration set, and clamp both rollers completely.	
____	____	____	7. Spike blood component unit bag port. Prime drip chamber and tubing with blood component.	
____	____	____	8. Spike 0.9% NaCl container with second spike. Keep roller clamp shut.	
____	____	____	9. Remove primary IV tubing from catheter hub, and cover end with sterile protector.	
____	____	____	10. Attach blood administration tubing to catheter hub, and secure with tape. The IV should be started into an 18- or 19-gauge catheter (if it is not already present).	
____	____	____	11. Open clamp to blood component. Open roller clamp below drip chamber and begin transfusion. Infuse blood slowly for first 15 minutes (10 drops per minute).	

PROCEDURE 29-8
Administering a Blood Transfusion (*Continued*)

Excellent	Satisfactory	Needs Practice	**Goal:** To replace blood volume or blood components lost through trauma, surgery, or a disease process; to prevent complications from transfusing incompatible blood products.	**Comments**
___ ___ ___			12. Observe and document client's condition during first 15 minutes, assessing for chilling, back pain, headache, nausea or vomiting, tachycardia, hypotension, tachypnea, or skin rash. *Note:* If any adverse reactions occur, close clamp to blood, open clamp to 0.9% NaCl, and notify physician immediately. Follow agency policy for laboratory notification and obtaining blood and urine specimens.	
___ ___ ___			13. If no adverse reactions occur after 15 minutes, regulate clamp to increase infusion according to physician's orders. A unit of red blood cells is usually administered over 2 to 4 hours. Observe the patient for signs and symptoms of transfusion reaction at least every 30 minutes throughout the transfusion. Obtain vital signs when observations warrant. Document observations, including the absence of any signs of transfusion reaction, in the medical record.	
___ ___ ___			14. When blood transfusion is complete, clamp roller to blood and open roller to 0.9% NaCl. Infuse until tubing is clear (usually no more than 50 mL of normal saline).	
___ ___ ___			15. Obtain and document vital signs.	
___ ___ ___			16. If second blood component unit is to be transfused, slow 0.9% NaCl to keep vein open until next unit is available. Follow verification procedure and vital sign monitoring for each unit.	
___ ___ ___			17. If transfusion orders are complete, disconnect the blood administration tubing from the IV catheter hub. Reconnect the primary IV solution and tubing and adjust to desired rate.	
___ ___ ___			18. Wash hands and document procedure.	

Procedure Checklists for Craven and Hirnle's Fundamentals of Nursing: Human Health and Function, 6th edition

Name _____ Date _____

Unit _____ Position _____

Instructor/Evaluator: _____ Position _____

Excellent	Satisfactory	Needs Practice	PROCEDURE 30-1 **Surgical Hand Scrub**	Comments
			Goal: To remove as many microorganisms from the hands as possible before a sterile procedure; to decrease the risk of infection for high-risk groups (e.g., newborns, transplant recipients).	
____	____	____	1. Remove rings. Apply surgical attire (scrubs, shoe cover, cap or hood, face mask, and protective eye wear).	
____	____	____	2. Turn on water using foot controls.	
____	____	____	3. Wash and rinse hands for the initial wash. Some alcohol-based surgical hand products have recently been developed that combine alcohol and antimicrobials with a prolonged activity against gram-negative and gram-positive organisms (Rothrock, 2007).	
____	____	____	4. Open disposable brush impregnated with anti-microbial soap and adjust water temperature to warm using water control lever.	
____	____	____	5. Wet hands and arms. Keep elbows bent so that hands remain higher than elbows. Water will flow down hands and off elbows.	
____	____	____	6. Use nail stick or cleaner to clean under nails of both hands.	
____	____	____	7. Wet scrub brush or apply antibacterial soap if not already impregnated in the brush. *Anatomic Timed Scrub.* Starting with the fingertips, scrub each anatomic area (nails, fingers each side and web space, palmar surface, dorsal surface, and forearm) for the designated amount of time according to agency policy (total usually around 5 minutes). Scrub vigorously using vertical strokes. Repeat with other hand. *Counted Brush Stroke Method.* Starting with the fingertips, scrub each anatomic area (nails, fingers each side and web space, palmar surface, dorsal surface, and forearm) for the designated number of strokes according to agency policy. Scrub vigorously using vertical strokes.	
____	____	____	8. Use anatomical timed scrub (usually around 5 minutes) or counted brush stroke method to scrub each anatomic area for the designated amount of time according to agency policy. Scrub	

PROCEDURE 30-1
Surgical Hand Scrub (*Continued*)

Excellent	Satisfactory	Needs Practice	**Goal:** To remove as many microorganisms from the hands as possible before a sterile procedure; to decrease the risk of infection for high-risk groups (e.g., newborns, transplant recipients).	Comments
			vigorously using vertical strokes. Repeat with other hand. — Start by scrubbing fingertips and nails — Scrub each side of fingers and web space — Scrub palmar surface — Scrub dorsal surface — Scrub exterior side of forearm — Scrub interior side of forearm	
___	___	___	9. Do not touch faucet, clothing, or other objects. Avoid splashing. Rinse hands thoroughly under warm running water, keeping hands elevated to allow water to drain off at the flexed elbow.	
___	___	___	10. Keep hands held upward to allow water to drip from the elbow. Dry with sterile towel.	

*Procedure Checklists for Craven and Hirnle's Fundamentals
of Nursing: Human Health and Function,* 6th edition

Name _____   Date _____

Unit _____   Position _____

Instructor/Evaluator: _____   Position _____

<table>
<tr><th>Excellent</th><th>Satisfactory</th><th>Needs Practice</th><th>PROCEDURE 30-2
Applying a Sterile Gown and Closed Gloving</th><th>Comments</th></tr>
<tr><td></td><td></td><td></td><td colspan="2">**Goal:** To apply attire necessary to safely carry out sterile procedures.</td></tr>
<tr><td>____</td><td>____</td><td>____</td><td>1. Locate all surgical attire (scrubs, shoe covers, cap or hood, face mask, and protective eye wear) and perform the surgical hand scrub as described in Procedure 30-1.</td><td></td></tr>
<tr><td></td><td></td><td></td><td>**Applying a Sterile Gown**</td><td></td></tr>
<tr><td>____</td><td>____</td><td>____</td><td>2. Grasp folded sterile gown at the neckline and step away from the sterile field. Allow gown to gently unfold, being careful that it does not touch the floor. The inside of the gown is toward the wearer. Slide arms in the sleeves until the fingers are at the end of the cuffs but not through the cuffs.</td><td></td></tr>
<tr><td>____</td><td>____</td><td>____</td><td>3. Have someone tie the back of the gown, taking care that only the ties are touched and not the sides or front of the gown.</td><td></td></tr>
<tr><td></td><td></td><td></td><td>**Closed Gloving**</td><td></td></tr>
<tr><td>____</td><td>____</td><td>____</td><td>4. With fingers still within the cuff of the gown, open the inner sterile glove package and pick up the first glove by the cuff, using your nondominant hand.</td><td></td></tr>
<tr><td>____</td><td>____</td><td>____</td><td>5. Position the glove with the fingers toward your body and the glove thumb side down, lying the glove over the cuff of the sterile gown. Grab both sides of the glove's cuff with both hands that still remain within the sleeves and cuff of the sterile gown. Stretch the entire glove over the stockinet cuff, being careful not to touch the edge of the stockinet cuff. Fingers remain within the cuff of the gown.</td><td></td></tr>
<tr><td>____</td><td>____</td><td>____</td><td>6. Work the fingers into the glove and pull the glove up over wrist with the nondominant hand that still remains within the cuff of the gown.</td><td></td></tr>
<tr><td>____</td><td>____</td><td>____</td><td>7. Use the sterile gloved hand to pick up the second glove, placing it over the stockinet cuff of the dominant hand and repeating the glove application process.</td><td></td></tr>
<tr><td>____</td><td>____</td><td>____</td><td>8. Adjust gloves for comfort and fit, taking care to keep gloved hands above waist level at all times.</td><td></td></tr>
</table>

Procedure Checklists for Craven and Hirnle's Fundamentals
of Nursing: Human Health and Function, 6th edition

Name _____   Date _____

Unit _____   Position _____

Instructor/Evaluator: _____   Position _____

Excellent	Satisfactory	Needs Practice	PROCEDURE 31-1 **Application of Restraints**	Comments
			Goal: To promote safety; to manage violent or self-destructive behavior that jeopardizes the immediate physical safety of the client, staff members, or others.	
____	____	____	**STEP 1** 1. Note the "front" and "back" of the restraint.	
____	____	____	**STEP 2** 1. Carefully apply the device and adjust properly so it maintains body alignment and ensures client comfort.	
____	____	____	2. Wrap the restraint around extremity with soft pad touching skin.	
____	____	____	3. Secure in place. 4. Ensure that two fingers can be inserted between the restraint and the client's wrist.	
____	____	____	**STEP 3** 1. Secure restraints designed for use in bed to the bed springs or frame, never to the mattress or the bed rails.	
____	____	____	**STEP 4** 1. Tie knots with appropriate hitches so they may be released quickly.	
____	____	____	**STEP 5** 1. Observe clients in restraints frequently, describing the client's behavior, the intervention used, and the client's response to the intervention. The client must be assessed face to face within 1 hour of application and frequently thereafter.	
____	____	____	2. Remove the restraints at least every 2 hours and more often if necessary. Allow for activities of daily living.	
____	____	____	**STEP 6** 1. Continue assessment even after a restraint is used, and discontinue use as soon as feasible. Restraint use should be considered a temporary solution to a situation.	
____	____	____	2. Clearly document in the client's record the medical reason for use of the restraint, the type selected, and the length of time for treatment.	

Procedure Checklists for Craven and Hirnle's Fundamentals of Nursing: Human Health and Function, 6th edition

Name _____ Date _____

Unit _____ Position _____

Instructor/Evaluator: _____ Position _____

PROCEDURE 33-1
Assisting With the Bath or Shower

Goal: To cleanse the skin, control body odors, and promote self-esteem; to stimulate circulation; to provide an opportunity to assess skin and physical mobility; to provide range-of-motion exercises for joints; to promote relaxation and comfort.

Excellent	Satisfactory	Needs Practice		Comments
——	——	——	1. Make sure the tub or shower is clean.	
——	——	——	2. Prepare bathroom by placing towel or disposable bathmat on floor by tub or shower.	
——	——	——	3. Accompany or transport client to the bathroom. Some clients may need to use a shower chair for transportation.	
——	——	——	4. Place "occupied" sign on door.	
——	——	——	5. Keep client covered with a bath blanket until water is ready.	
——	——	——	6. Fill bathtub halfway with warm water (105°F, 40.6°C). Test water or have client test water. If the client is taking a shower, turn on shower and adjust water temperature.	
——	——	——	7. Help client into shower or tub, providing necessary assistance.	
——	——	——	8. Instruct the client in use of safety bars and call bell signal. Client may prefer to sit in shower chair to prevent fatigue.	
——	——	——	9. If the client is unable to shower independently, stay with the client at all times. (Two nurses may be necessary for some clients.) Use handheld shower to wet client. Wash client with soap and washcloth using long, firm strokes.	
——	——	——	10. If client is showering or bathing independently, check on client within 15 minutes. Wash any areas he or she could not reach.	
——	——	——	11. Assist with drying. Help client out of tub or shower. If client is unsteady, drain water before helping client out of tub.	
——	——	——	12. Assist client with dressing and grooming.	
——	——	——	13. Help client to room. Return to bathroom and clean tub or shower according to agency policy. Discard soiled linen. Place "unoccupied" sign on door.	

Procedure Checklists for Craven and Hirnle's Fundamentals of Nursing: Human Health and Function, 6th edition

Name _____ Date _____

Unit _____ Position _____

Instructor/Evaluator: _____ Position _____

Excellent	Satisfactory	Needs Practice	PROCEDURE 33-2 **Bathing a Client in Bed**	Comments
			Goal: Same as Procedure 33-1.	
___	___	___	1. Close curtains around bed or shut room door. 2. Help client use bedpan, urinal, or commode if needed.	
___	___	___	3. Close window and door to decrease drafts. 4. Wash your hands. 5. Raise bed to high position. Lock up side rail on opposite side of bed from your work.	
___	___	___	6. Remove top sheet and bedspread, then place bath blanket on client. Help client move closer to you, and remove client's gown. If client has an IV line, remove gown from arm, lower IV container, and slide it through gown with tubing. Rehang IV container, and check flow rate. If top linen is to be reused, place it on back of chair; otherwise place it in laundry bag.	
___	___	___	7. Lay towel across client's chest. 8. Remove first cloth from bag bath packet. *OR* Wet washcloth and fold around your finger to make a mitt.	
___	___	___	a. Fold washcloth in thirds.	
___	___	___	b. Straighten washcloth to take out wrinkles. c. Fold washcloth over to fit hand. d. Tuck loose ends under edge of washcloth on palm.	
___	___	___	9. Cleanse eyes with water only, wiping from inner to outer canthus. Use separate corner of mitt for each eye.	
___	___	___	10. Determine if client would like soap used on face. Wash face, neck, and ears. Liquid nondetergent cleansing agents are available in many institutions to mix directly into bath water. These products are nondrying and need not be rinsed from the skin. *or* Use first disposable cloth to cleanse face.	
___	___	___	11. Fold bath blanket off arm away from you. Place towel lengthwise under arm. Wash, rinse, and dry the arm using long, firm strokes from the fingers toward the axilla. Wash axilla. Place folded towel	

Excellent	Satisfactory	Needs Practice	PROCEDURE 33-2 **Bathing a Client in Bed (*Continued*)**	
			Goal: Same as Procedure 33-1.	**Comments**

and water basin on client's bed. Soak client's hand, wash and rinse.

or

Continue to use disposable bag bath cloths as directed on the package, cleansing parts of the body.

____ ____ ____ 12. Repeat for hand and arm nearest you.

____ ____ ____ 13. Apply deodorant or powder according to client's preferences. Avoid excessive use of powder or inhalation of powder.

____ ____ ____ 14. Assess bath water temperature and change water if necessary. Side rails should be up.

____ ____ ____ 15. Place bath towel over chest. Fold bath blanket down to below umbilicus.

____ ____ ____ 16. Lift bath towel off chest, and bathe chest and abdomen with cloth using long, firm strokes. Give special attention to skin under the breasts and any other skin folds if client is overweight. Rinse and dry well. Apply a light dusting of bath powder under the breasts or between skin folds.

____ ____ ____ 17. Help client don a clean gown.

____ ____ ____ 18. Expose leg away from you by folding over bath blanket. Be careful to keep perineum covered.

____ ____ ____ 19. Lift leg, and place bath towel lengthwise under leg. Wash, rinse, and dry leg using long, firm strokes from ankle to thigh.

____ ____ ____ 20. Wash feet. Rinse and dry well. Pay special attention to space between toes.

____ ____ ____ 21. Repeat for other leg and foot.

____ ____ ____ 22. Assess bath water for warmth. Change water if necessary.

____ ____ ____ 23. Assist client to side-lying position. Apply gloves. Place bath towel along side of back and buttocks to protect linen. Wash, rinse, and dry back and buttocks. Give a backrub with lotion.

____ ____ ____ 24. Assist client to supine position. Assess if client can wash genitals and perineal area independently. If client needs help, drape with blanket so that only genitals are exposed. Don disposable, clean gloves. Using fresh water and a new cloth, wash, rinse, and dry genitalia and perineum (see text for instructions).

____ ____ ____ 25. Complete care according to client's preference. Apply powder, lotion, cologne. Assist with hair and mouth care. Make bed with clean linen.

____ ____ ____ 26. Clean equipment and return to appropriate storage area. Wash your hands.

*Procedure Checklists for Craven and Hirnle's Fundamentals
of Nursing: Human Health and Function*, 6th edition

Name _____   Date _____

Unit _____   Position _____

Instructor/Evaluator: _____   Position _____

Excellent	Satisfactory	Needs Practice	PROCEDURE 33-3 **Massaging the Back**	Comments
			Goal: To stimulate circulation to the skin; to relieve muscle tension; to promote comfort and relaxation.	
___	___	___	1. Help client to side-lying or prone position.	
___	___	___	2. Expose back, shoulders, upper arms, and sacral area. Cover remainder of body with bath blanket.	
___	___	___	3. Wash hands in warm water. Warm lotion by holding container under running warm water.	
___	___	___	4. Pour small amount of lotion into palms.	
___	___	___	5. Begin massage in sacral area with circular motion. Move hands upward to shoulders, massaging over scapulae in smooth, firm strokes. Without removing hands from skin, continue in smooth strokes to upper arms and down sides of back to iliac crest. Continue for 3 to 5 minutes.	
___	___	___	6. While massaging, assess for broken skin areas and whitish or reddened areas that do not disappear. Do not apply pressure over areas of breakdown or redness.	
___	___	___	7. If additional stimulation is desired, nurse can use petrissage (kneading) over the shoulders and gluteal area and tapotement (tapping) up and down the spine.	
___	___	___	8. End massage with long, continuous, stroking movements.	
___	___	___	9. Pat excess lubricant dry with towel. Retie client's gown, and assist to comfortable position.	
___	___	___	10. Wash your hands.	

Procedure Checklists for Craven and Hirnle's Fundamentals
of Nursing: Human Health and Function, 6th edition

Name _____ Date _____

Unit _____ Position _____

Instructor/Evaluator: _____ Position _____

Excellent	Satisfactory	Needs Practice	PROCEDURE 33-4 **Performing Foot and Hand Care**	Comments
			Goal: To maintain skin integrity; to provide for client's comfort and sense of well-being; to maintain foot function and ability to ambulate; to encourage self-care.	
___	___	___	1. Wash your hands.	
___	___	___	2. Identify client and help to chair if possible. Elevate head of bed for bedridden client.	
___	___	___	3. Fill washbasin with warm water (100°–104°F; 37.7°–40°C). Place waterproof pad under basin. Soak client's hands or feet in basin. Clients with diabetes may soak their feet for a short period of time, provided that the water is not too hot.	
___	___	___	4. Place call bell within reach. Allow hands or feet to soak for 10 to 20 minutes.	
___	___	___	5. Dry the hand or foot that has been soaking. Rewarm water, and allow other extremity to soak while you work on the softened nails.	
___	___	___	6. Gently clean under nails with cuticle stick. If nails are thickened and yellow, client may have a fungal infection. Wear disposable gloves and eye protection.	
___	___	___	7. Beginning with large toe or thumb, clip nail straight across. Shape nail with file. File rather than cut nails of clients with diabetes or circulatory problems.	
___	___	___	8. Push back cuticle gently with cuticle stick.	
___	___	___	9. Repeat procedure with other nails.	
___	___	___	10. Rinse foot or hand in warm water.	
___	___	___	11. Dry thoroughly with towel, especially between digits.	
___	___	___	12. Apply lotion to hands or feet. Do not apply lotion between the toes of the client with diabetes.	
___	___	___	13. Help client to comfortable position.	
___	___	___	14. Remove and dispose of equipment.	
___	___	___	15. Wash your hands.	

Procedure Checklists for Craven and Hirnle's Fundamentals
of Nursing: Human Health and Function, 6th edition

Name _____   Date _____

Unit _____   Position _____

Instructor/Evaluator: _____   Position _____

PROCEDURE 33-5
Shampooing Hair of a Bedridden Client

Excellent	Satisfactory	Needs Practice	**Goal:** To cleanse hair and scalp; to promote comfort and self-esteem; to apply medication to scalp and hair.	Comments
___	___	___	1. Place waterproof pads under client's head and shoulders, and remove pillow.	
___	___	___	2. Raise bed to highest position.	
___	___	___	3. Remove any pins from hair. Comb and brush hair thoroughly.	
___	___	___	4. Adjust bed to flat position. Place shampooing basin under head. Place bath towel around shoulders and folded washcloth where neck rests on basin.	
___	___	___	5. Fold bed linens down to waist. Cover upper body with bath blanket.	
___	___	___	6. Place waste basket with plastic bag under spout of shampoo basin on a chair or table at the bedside.	
___	___	___	7. Using water pitcher, wet hair thoroughly with warm water (approximately 110°F or 43.3°C). Check temperature by placing small amount of water on your wrist.	
___	___	___	8. Apply small amount of shampoo. Before shampooing, use hydrogen peroxide to dissolve matted blood in hair. Peroxide normally feels bubbly and warm. Reassure client that it will not bleach hair.	
___	___	___	9. Massage scalp with fingertips while making shampoo lather. Start at hairline and work toward neck.	
___	___	___	10. Rinse hair with warm water. Reapply shampoo and repeat massage.	
___	___	___	11. Rinse hair thoroughly with warm water. Clean hair "squeaks" when rubbed between fingers.	
___	___	___	12. Apply small amount of conditioner per client request. Rinse well.	
___	___	___	13. Squeeze excess moisture from hair. Wrap bath towel around hair. Rub to dry hair and scalp. Use second towel if necessary.	
___	___	___	14. Remove equipment and wet towels from bed. Place dry towel over client's shoulders.	
___	___	___	15. Dry hair with hair dryer if necessary. Comb and style.	
___	___	___	16. Help client to comfortable position.	
___	___	___	17. Dispose of soiled equipment and linen.	

Excellent	Satisfactory	Needs Practice	

Shampooing Hair of a Bedridden Client (*Continued*)

Goal: To cleanse hair and scalp; to promote comfort and self-esteem; to apply medication to scalp and hair.

Comments

Variation for Using a Dry Shampoo Cap

1. Spread towel across client's chest and place shampoo cap on client.
2. Massage scalp so that dry shampoo is evenly distributed.
3. Wait 1 to 3 minutes for shampoo to fully saturate hair.
4. Remove and discard shampoo cap.
5. Use clean towel to dry client's hair.
6. Groom and style client's hair.

Procedure Checklists for Craven and Hirnle's Fundamentals
of Nursing: Human Health and Function, 6th edition

Name _____   Date _____

Unit _____   Position _____

Instructor/Evaluator: _____   Position _____

PROCEDURE 33-6
Providing Oral Care

Goal: To cleanse tooth surfaces to prevent odor and caries; to maintain hydrated, intact oral mucosa; to promote self-esteem and comfort.

Excellent	Satisfactory	Needs Practice		Comments
___	___	___	1. Wash your hands.	
___	___	___	2. Close bedside curtains or room door, identify client, and explain procedure.	
___	___	___	3. Help client to a sitting position. If client cannot sit, help to a side-lying position.	
___	___	___	4. Place towel under client's chin.	
___	___	___	5. Moisten toothbrush with water. Apply small amount of toothpaste. If client is anticoagulated or has a clotting disorder, use a very soft toothbrush or a sponge-ended swab to prevent gum bleeding.	
___	___	___	6. Hand toothbrush to client or don disposable gloves and brush client's teeth as follows:	
___	___	___	a. Hold toothbrush at a 45-degree angle to the gum line.	
___	___	___	b. Using short, vibrating motions, brush from the gum line to the crown of each tooth. Repeat until outside and inside of teeth and gums are cleaned.	
___	___	___	c. Cleanse biting surfaces by brushing with a back-and-forth stroke.	
___	___	___	d. Brush the tongue lightly. Avoid stimulating the gag reflex.	
___	___	___	7. Have client rinse mouth thoroughly with water and spit into emesis basin.	
___	___	___	8. Remove emesis basin, set aside, and dry client's mouth with washcloth.	
___	___	___	9. Floss client's teeth.	
___	___	___	a. Cut 10-inch piece of dental floss. Wind ends of floss around middle finger of each hand.	
___	___	___	b. Using index fingers to stretch the floss, move the floss up and down around and between lower teeth. Start at the back lower teeth and work around to the other side.	
___	___	___	c. Using thumb and index fingers to stretch the floss, repeat procedure on upper teeth.	
___	___	___	d. Have client rinse mouth thoroughly and spit into emesis basin.	
___	___	___	10. Remove and dispose of supplies. Help client to comfortable position.	
___	___	___	11. Wash your hands.	

PROCEDURE 33-6

Providing Oral Care (*Continued*)

Goal: To cleanse tooth surfaces to prevent odor and caries; to maintain hydrated, intact oral mucosa; to promote self-esteem and comfort.

Excellent	Satisfactory	Needs Practice		Comments

Variation for the Unconscious Client

1. Gather equipment.
2. Place client in a side-lying position.
3. Place towel or waterproof pad under client's chin.
4. Place emesis basin against client's mouth or have suction catheter positioned to remove secretions from mouth.
5. Use padded tongue blade to open teeth gently. Leave in place between the back molars. Never put your fingers in an unconscious client's mouth.
6. Brush teeth and gums as directed previously, using toothbrush or soft sponge-ended swab. Cleanse oral cavity using toothette.
7. Use a small bulb syringe or syringe without needle to rinse oral cavity. Swab or use oral suction to remove pooled secretions.
8. Apply thin layer of petroleum jelly to lips to prevent drying or cracking.

Procedure Checklists for Craven and Hirnle's Fundamentals of Nursing: Human Health and Function, 6th edition

Name _____   Date _____

Unit _____   Position _____

Instructor/Evaluator: _____   Position _____

Excellent	Satisfactory	Needs Practice	PROCEDURE 33-7 **Using a Bedpan**	Comments
			Goal: To provide a means for elimination for clients who are confined to bed or unable to get to the bathroom or bedside commode independently or safely.	

Placing the Bedpan

___	___	___	1. Wash your hands. Don clean gloves.
___	___	___	2. Close curtain around bed or shut door.
___	___	___	3. Position and lock side rail up on opposite side of bed from which you will work.
___	___	___	4. Raise bed to height appropriate for nurse.
___	___	___	5. For client who can raise buttocks and assist with procedure:
			a. Fold top linen down on your side to expose the client's hips. (Client in photographs is exposed for better visualization of procedure.)
___	___	___	b. Have client flex knees and lift buttocks. Slide waterproof pad under client.
___	___	___	c. Assist client by placing your hand under sacrum, elbow on mattress, and lifting as a lever. Slide rounded, smooth rim of regular bedpan under client. If using a fracture pan, slide narrow, flat end under buttocks.
___	___	___	6. For client unable to assist by raising buttocks:
___	___	___	a. Lower head of bed to flat position.
___	___	___	b. Fold top bed linens down to expose client minimally.
___	___	___	c. Help client to roll to side-lying position.
___	___	___	d. Place bedpan against buttocks and tucked down against mattress. Hold firmly in place and roll client onto back as bedpan is positioned under buttocks.
___	___	___	7. Cover client with linen. Place call bell and toilet paper within reach.
___	___	___	8. Raise head of bed 45 to 80 degrees unless contraindicated.
___	___	___	9. Lower bed to lowest position. Place side rails up if indicated.
___	___	___	10. Wash your hands. Allow client to be alone.

Removing the Bedpan

___	___	___	11. Answer call bell promptly.
___	___	___	12. Place soap, wet washcloth, and towel at bedside.

PROCEDURE 33-7
Using a Bedpan (*Continued*)

Goal: To provide a means for elimination for clients who are confined to bed or unable to get to the bathroom or bedside commode independently or safely.

Excellent	Satisfactory	Needs Practice		Comments

13. Raise bed to appropriate working height for nurse.
14. Fold back top linens to expose client minimally.
15. Put on disposable clean gloves.
16. Assess if client can wipe perineal area. If not, wipe area with several layers of toilet tissue. If specimen is to be measured or collected, dispose of soiled toilet tissue in separate receptacle, not bedpan. For female clients, wipe from urethra toward anus.
17. For client who can raise buttocks and assist with procedure:
    a. Lower head of bed.
    b. Have client flex knees and lift buttocks. Assist client by placing one hand under sacrum and supporting bedpan with other hand to prevent spillage. Remove bedpan and place on bedside chair.
    c. Offer soap, warm water, washcloth, and towel for client to wash hands or perineal area.
18. For client unable to assist by raising buttocks:
    a. Lower head of bed to flat position.
    b. Fold top linen down to expose client minimally.
    c. Help client to roll off bedpan and onto side. Use one hand to stabilize bedpan during turning to prevent spillage.
    d. Wipe anal area with tissue. Wash perineum with soap and warm water. Pat dry.
19. Assist client to comfortable position.
20. Cover bedpan and remove from bedside. Obtain specimen if required. Empty and clean bedpan, and return it to bedside.
21. Remove and discard gloves. Wash your hands.
22. Spray air freshener if necessary to control odor, unless contraindicated (client with respiratory conditions, allergies).

Procedure Checklists for Craven and Hirnle's Fundamentals
of Nursing: Human Health and Function, 6th edition

Name _____   Date _____

Unit _____   Position _____

Instructor/Evaluator: _____   Position _____

Excellent	Satisfactory	Needs Practice	PROCEDURE 33-8 **Making an Occupied Bed**	Comments
			Goal: To provide clean linen for client who is unable to get out of bed; to promote comfort.	
— — —	— — —	— — —	1. Wash your hands. 2. Assemble equipment on bedside table or chair. Do not place on another client's bed. 3. Close room door or bedside curtains. 4. Lock up side rails on side of bed opposite from where you stack the clean linen. 5. Raise bed to comfortable working position. Lower side rail on your side of bed. 6. Loosen all top linen from foot of bed. Remove top linen and bedspread or blanket separately. Without shaking, fold each piece and place over back of chair if it is to be reused. If it is soiled, hold it away from your uniform and place in linen bag. 7. Leave top sheet on client or cover client with a bath blanket; if using bath blanket remove top sheet from under bath blanket and discard top sheet. (A bath blanket does not appear in photos, for better visualization.) 8. Loosen the bottom sheet on your side. Lower head of bed to flat position. If client cannot tolerate flat position, lower head of bed as far as client can tolerate. 9. Help client to roll onto side facing away from you. Client may grasp side rail to assist. Additional personnel may be needed to assist with client positioning. Adjust pillow under head. 10. Tightly fanfold soiled linens. Tuck under buttocks, back, and shoulders. Do not fanfold mattress pad unless it is soiled. **For Flat Bottom Sheet** 11. Unfold lengthwise so bottom edge is even with end of mattress and vertical center crease is at center of bed. 12. Bring sheet's bottom edge over mattress sides and fanfold top of sheet toward center of mattress and place next to client. Tuck top edge of sheet under mattress. Miter top corner on your side.	

Excellent	Satisfactory	Needs Practice	PROCEDURE 33-8 **Making an Occupied Bed (*Continued*)**	Comments
			Goal: To provide clean linen for client who is unable to get out of bed; to promote comfort.	
___	___	___	a. Grasp side edge of sheet about 18 inches down from mattress top.	
___	___	___	b. Lay sheet on top of mattress to form a triangular, flat fold.	
___	___	___	c. Tuck sheet hanging loose below mattress under mattress without pulling on the triangular fold.	
___	___	___	d. Pick up triangular fold, and place it over side of the mattress.	
___	___	___	e. Tuck this loose portion of sheet under the mattress.	
___	___	___	13. Tuck remaining portion of sheet under mattress. Proceed to Step 15.	

For Fitted Sheet

Excellent	Satisfactory	Needs Practice		Comments
___	___	___	14. Secure the top and bottom elastic edges over the side of the mattress nearest you. Fanfold top of sheet toward center of mattress and place next to client.	
___	___	___	15. Place draw sheet on bed with center fold at center of bed. Position sheet so it will extend from the client's back to below the buttocks. Fanfold the top edge and place next to client. Tuck excess under mattress. Some agencies use a cloth waterproof pad instead of a draw sheet.	
___	___	___	16. Position top sheet and draw sheet under soiled sheets.	
___	___	___	17. Lock up side rails on your side and move to other side of bed.	
___	___	___	18. Lower side rail. Help client to roll over folds of linen onto his or her other side. You may need additional help if client is unable to move easily. Move pillow under client's head.	
___	___	___	19. Remove soiled linen by folding into a square or bundle with soiled side turned in. Place in linen bag.	
___	___	___	20. Grasp edge of fanfolded bottom sheet and pull from under the client.	
___	___	___	21. If using flat sheet, tuck top of sheet under top of mattress and miter top corner. Pull bottom sheet tight and tuck excess linen under mattress from top to bottom. If using fitted sheet, secure elastic corners at the head and foot of mattress.	
___	___	___	22. Unfold draw sheet by grasping at center. Pull draw sheet taut and smooth. Tuck excess tightly under mattress. Tuck the middle first, then the top, and finally the bottom.	
___	___	___	23. Help client to center of bed.	

PROCEDURE 33-8
Making an Occupied Bed (*Continued*)

Excellent	Satisfactory	Needs Practice	

Goal: To provide clean linen for client who is unable to get out of bed; to promote comfort.

Comments

24. Raise side rail if necessary and move to side of bed where remainder of linen is stored.
25. Place top sheet over client with center crease lengthwise at center of bed with seam side up. Unfold sheet from head to toe.
26. Have client grasp top edge of clean top sheet. Remove bath blanket or soiled top linen by pulling from beneath clean top sheet. Smooth sheet, with excess falling over bottom edge of mattress.
27. Discard in linen bag.
28. Place top sheet on bed with vertical center fold at center of bed. Unfold sheet with seams facing out and top edge even with top of mattress. Smooth sheet, with excess falling over bottom edge of mattress.
29. Spread blanket or bedspread evenly over bed. Miter the bottom corner, using all layers of linen (sheet, blanket, bedspread). Leave sides untucked. Move to opposite side of bed and repeat.
30. Standing at bottom of bed, grasp top covers about 10 inches from bottom of mattress. Loosen linen slightly by pulling on top covers or forming a pleat.
31. Put on clean pillowcases:
    a. Grasp center of pillowcase with one hand on seamed end.
    b. Gather case, turning it inside out over the hand holding it.
    c. With same hand, grasp middle of one end of pillow.
    d. Pull case over pillow with free hand.
    e. Adjust case so corners fit over pillow.
32. Place pillows in center at head of bed.
33. Ensure that call bell is within client's reach, and lower bed.
34. Arrange the bedside table, night stand, and personal items within easy reach.
35. Discard soiled linens and wash your hands.

Procedure Checklists for Craven and Hirnle's Fundamentals of Nursing: Human Health and Function, 6th edition

Name _____ Date _____

Unit _____ Position _____

Instructor/Evaluator: _____ Position _____

Excellent	Satisfactory	Needs Practice	PROCEDURE 34-1 **Using Body Mechanics to Move Clients**	Comments
			Goal: To prevent injury to the nurse's musculoskeletal system; to prevent injury to the client during transfer.	
___	___	___	1. Plan movement before doing it.	
___	___	___	a. Always lock wheels on bed, stretcher, or wheelchair.	
___	___	___	b. Allow client to assist during move.	
___	___	___	c. Use mechanical aids (e.g., transfer belts, mechanical lifts, slide boards, body mobilizers) or additional personnel to move heavy clients.	
___	___	___	d. When possible, slide, push, or pull client rather than lifting and carrying.	
___	___	___	e. Tighten abdominal and gluteal muscles before lifting or moving client.	
___	___	___	f. Use smooth, rhythmic, coordinated motions.	
___	___	___	g. If another person is assisting, plan your movements before beginning.	
___	___	___	2. Begin all movements with body aligned and balanced.	
___	___	___	a. Face client to be moved, and plan to pivot your entire body without twisting your back.	
___	___	___	b. Place both feet flat on floor; position your feet and shins alongside the client's feet and shins; bend knees slightly with one foot slightly in front of the other or one step apart.	
___	___	___	c. Bend knees to lower center of gravity toward client to be moved.	
___	___	___	3. Grasp transfer belt using an underhand grip or pass your arms under the client's arms, placing your hands on the client's upper back. Assist client to stand.	
			4. When possible, elevate adjustable beds to waist level and lower side rails.	
___	___	___	5. Carry objects close to body, and stand as close as possible to work area.	

Procedure Checklists for Craven and Hirnle's Fundamentals
of Nursing: Human Health and Function, 6th edition

Name _____   Date _____

Unit _____   Position _____

Instructor/Evaluator: _____   Position _____

Excellent	Satisfactory	Needs Practice	PROCEDURE 34-2 **Positioning a Client in Bed**	Comments
			Goal: To maintain proper body alignment; to maintain skin integrity and prevent deformities of the musculoskeletal system; to provide comfort; to maintain optimal position for ventilation and lung expansion.	
___	___	___	1. Identify client and any positioning or mobility restrictions. Explain procedure and rationale to client.	
___	___	___	2. Lower head of bed as flat as client can tolerate. Raise level of bed to comfortable working height.	
___	___	___	3. Remove all pillows from under client. Leave one at head of bed.	
			Moving a Client Up in Bed (One Nurse)	
___	___	___	1. Instruct client to bend legs and put feet flat on bed.	
___	___	___	2. Place your feet in broad stance with one foot in front of the other. Flex your knees and use your thighs.	
___	___	___	3. Place one arm under client's shoulders and one arm under thighs. Keep head up and back straight. Ask client to fold the arms across chest, if able. Have client lift head and place chin on chest.	
___	___	___	4. Rock back and forth on front and back legs to count of three. On third count, have client push with feet as you lift and assist the client up in bed.	
___	___	___	5. Elevate head of bed and place pillows under head. Raise side rails and lower bed to lowest level.	
			Moving Helpless Client Up in Bed (Two Nurses)	
___	___	___	1. One nurse stands on each side of bed with legs positioned for wide base of support and one foot slightly in front of the other.	
___	___	___	2. Each nurse rolls up and grasps edges of turn sheet close to client's shoulders and buttocks.	
___	___	___	3. Flex knees and hips. Tighten abdominal and gluteal muscles and keep back straight.	
___	___	___	4. Rock back and forth on front and back legs to count of three. On third count, both nurses shift weight to front leg as they simultaneously lift client toward head of bed.	
___	___	___	5. Elevate head of bed and place pillows under client's head. Adjust other positioning pillows as necessary. Put up side rails and lower bed to lowest level.	

PROCEDURE 34-2
Positioning a Client in Bed (*Continued*)

Goal: To maintain proper body alignment; to maintain skin integrity and prevent deformities of the musculoskeletal system; to provide comfort; to maintain optimal position for ventilation and lung expansion.

Excellent	Satisfactory	Needs Practice		Comments

Positioning Client in Side-Lying Position

1. Elevate and lock side rail on side client will face when turned.
2. Using draw sheet, move client to the edge of the bed, opposite the side on which he or she will be turned.
3. Place arm that client will turn toward away from his or her body. Fold other arm across chest.
4. Flex client's knee that will not be next to mattress after turn. Have client reach toward side rail with opposite arm.
5. Assume a broad stance with knees slightly flexed.
6. Using draw sheet, gently pull client over on side.
7. Align client properly then place pillows behind back and under head.
8. Pull shoulder blade forward and out from under client. Support client's upper arm with pillow.
9. Place pillow lengthwise between client's legs from thighs to foot.
10. Cover client with top linen and blanket. Elevate head of bed. Put up side rails and lower bed to lower level.

Logrolling

1. Obtain assistance.
2. Nurses stand with feet apart, one foot slightly ahead of the other. Flex knees and hips.
3. Use one pillow to support client's head during and after turn. Instruct client to fold arms over chest and keep body stiff. Roll draw sheet toward client.
4. Place pillows between client's legs.
5. Reach across client and support head, thorax, trunk, and legs. On count of three, roll client in one coordinated movement to lateral position.
6. Support client in alignment with pillows as described in "Positioning Client in Side-Lying Position" above. Clients with suspected or known cervical spinal injuries should wear cervical collars.

Procedure Checklists for Craven and Hirnle's Fundamentals
of Nursing: Human Health and Function, 6th edition

Name _____   Date _____
Unit _____   Position _____
Instructor/Evaluator: _____   Position _____

Excellent	Satisfactory	Needs Practice	PROCEDURE 34-3 **Providing Range-of-Motion Exercises** **Goal:** To maintain joint mobility; to improve or maintain muscle strength; to prevent muscle atrophy and contractures.	Comments
—	—	—	1. Identify client and client's movement limitations. Explain procedure and purpose to client.	
—	—	—	2. Position client on back with head of bed as flat as possible. Elevate bed to comfortable working height.	
—	—	—	3. Stand on side of bed where joints are to be exercised. Uncover only the limb to be exercised.	
—	—	—	4. Refer to Table 34-1 for illustrations of normal movement for each joint. Perform exercises slowly and gently, providing support by holding areas proximal and distal to the joint. Often, this can be done while providing hygiene.	
—	—	—	5. Repeat each exercise five times. Discontinue or decrease ROM if client complains of discomfort or muscle spasm.	
—	—	—	6. Neck:	
—	—	—	a. Move chin to chest.	
—	—	—	b. Return head to upright position.	
—	—	—	c. Tilt head toward each shoulder.	
—	—	—	d. Move chin toward each shoulder.	
—	—	—	e. Rotate head in circular motion.	
—	—	—	f. Return head to erect position.	
—	—	—	7. Shoulder:	
—	—	—	a. Raise client's arm from side to above head.	
—	—	—	b. Abduct and rotate shoulder by raising arm above head with palm up.	
—	—	—	c. Adduct shoulder by moving arm across body as far as possible.	
—	—	—	d. Rotate shoulder internally and externally by flexing elbow and moving forearm so the palm touches mattress; then reverse the motion so that back of client's hand touches mattress.	
—	—	—	e. Move shoulder in a full circle.	
—	—	—	8. Elbow:	
—	—	—	a. Bend elbow so that forearm moves toward shoulder.	
—	—	—	b. Hyperextend elbow as far as possible.	
—	—	—	9. Wrist and hand:	
—	—	—	a. Rotate lower arm and hand so palm is up.	
—	—	—	b. Rotate lower arm and hand so palm is down.	

Excellent	Satisfactory	Needs Practice	

PROCEDURE 34-3
Providing Range-of-Motion Exercises (*Continued*)

Goal: To maintain joint mobility; to improve or maintain muscle strength; to prevent muscle atrophy and contractures.

Comments

Excellent	Satisfactory	Needs Practice	Steps
___	___	___	c. Move hand toward inner aspect of forearm.
___	___	___	d. Return hand to neutral position.
___	___	___	e. Bend dorsal surface of hand backward.
___	___	___	f. Abduct wrist by bending toward thumb.
___	___	___	g. Adduct wrist by bending toward fifth finger.
___	___	___	h. Make a fist; extend the fingers.
___	___	___	i. Spread fingers apart, then together.
___	___	___	j. Move thumb across hand to base of fifth finger.
			10. Hip and knee:
___	___	___	a. Lift leg and bend knee toward chest. Return leg to straightened position.
___	___	___	b. Abduct and adduct leg, moving leg laterally away from body. Return leg to medial position and try to extend it beyond the midpoint.
___	___	___	c. Internally and externally rotate hip by turning leg inward, then outward.
___	___	___	d. Take special care to support joints of larger limbs.
			11. Ankle and foot:
___	___	___	a. Dorsiflex foot by moving it so toes point upward.
___	___	___	b. Plantarflex by moving foot so toes point downward.
___	___	___	c. Curl toes down, then extend.
___	___	___	d. Spread toes apart, then bring together.
___	___	___	e. Invert by turning sole of foot medially.
___	___	___	f. Evert by turning sole of foot laterally.
___	___	___	12. Move to other side of bed and repeat exercises.
___	___	___	13. Reposition client comfortably.
___	___	___	14. Document ROM.

Procedure Checklists for Craven and Hirnle's Fundamentals of Nursing: Human Health and Function, 6th edition

Name _____ Date _____

Unit _____ Position _____

Instructor/Evaluator: _____ Position _____

Excellent	Satisfactory	Needs Practice		Comments
			PROCEDURE 34-4 **Assisting With Ambulation**	
			Goal: To promote safe ambulation free of falls or injury; to increase muscle strength and joint mobility; to prevent complications of immobility; to promote self-esteem and independence.	
___	___	___	1. Identify client. Explain procedure and purpose of ambulation to client. Decide together how far and where to walk.	
___	___	___	2. Place bed in lowest position.	
			3. Assist client to sitting position on side of bed. Assess for dizziness. Obtain orthostatic vital signs if complaints are present. Allow client to remain in this position until he or she feels secure.	
___	___	___	4. Help client with clothing and footwear.	
			One Nurse	
___	___	___	1. Wrap transfer belt around client's waist (optional according to previous assessment).	
___	___	___	2. Assist client to standing position and assess client's balance. Return client to bed or transfer to chair if he or she is very weak or unsteady. Be sure client does not grasp your neck for support but places his or her hands around your shoulders or at your waist.	
___	___	___	3. Assess client position when grasping cane. The handle of the cane should be level with the greater trochanter and should allow approximately 15 degrees of flexion at the elbow.	
___	___	___	4. Position yourself behind client while supporting him or her by waist or transfer belt.	
			5. Take several steps forward with client. Assess strength and balance. Encourage client to use good posture and to look ahead, not down at feet.	
___	___	___	6. Ambulate for planned distance or time. If client becomes weak or dizzy, return client to bed or assist to chair.	
___	___	___	7. If the client begins to fall, place your feet wide apart with one foot in front. Support the client by pulling his or her weight backward against your body. Lower gently to floor, protecting head.	

PROCEDURE 34-4
Assisting With Ambulation (*Continued*)

Goal: To promote safe ambulation free of falls or injury; to increase muscle strength and joint mobility; to prevent complications of immobility; to promote self-esteem and independence.

Excellent	Satisfactory	Needs Practice		Comments

Two Nurses

1. Assist client to sitting position as described.
2. Assist client to standing position with one nurse on each side.
3. One nurse grasps the transfer belt to support the client. The other nurse may carry and manage equipment.
4. Walk with client using slow, even steps. Assess strength and balance. Encourage client to look forward rather than down at floor.

Using a Walker

1. Assist client to standing position. Have client keep one hand on the arm of the chair or bed while she or he assumes an upright posture.
2. Have client grasp walker handles. Client moves walker ahead 6 to 8 inches placing all four feet of walker on floor. Client moves forward to walker.
3. Nurse should walk closely behind and slightly to side of client. Use a transfer belt if the client is not steady or is at risk for falling.
4. Repeat above sequence until walk is complete.

Procedure Checklists for Craven and Hirnle's Fundamentals
of Nursing: Human Health and Function, 6th edition

Name _____   Date _____

Unit _____   Position _____

Instructor/Evaluator: _____   Position _____

Excellent	Satisfactory	Needs Practice	PROCEDURE 34-5 **Helping Clients With Crutchwalking**	Comments
			Goal: To increase client's level of activity after musculo-skeletal injury; to assist client to walk safely with crutches using the least amount of energy.	
			Four-Point Gait	
___	___	___	1. Client stands erect, face forward in tripod position. Client places crutch tips 6 inches in front of feet and 6 inches to side of each foot.	
___	___	___	2. Client moves right crutch forward 6 inches.	
___	___	___	3. Client moves left foot forward to level of right crutch.	
___	___	___	4. Client moves left crutch forward 4 to 6 inches.	
___	___	___	5. Client moves right foot forward to level of left crutch.	
			6. Repeat sequence.	
			Three-Point Gait	
___	___	___	1. Beginning in the tripod position, client moves both crutches and affected leg forward.	
___	___	___	2. Client moves stronger leg forward.	
			3. Repeat sequence.	
			Two-Point Gait	
___	___	___	1. Beginning in the tripod position, client moves left crutch and right foot forward.	
___	___	___	2. Client moves right crutch and left foot forward.	
			3. Repeat sequence.	
			Swing-To Gait	
___	___	___	1. Client forms tripod position and moves both crutches forward.	
___	___	___	2. Client lifts legs and swings to crutches, supporting body weight on crutches.	
			Swing-Through Gait	
___	___	___	1. Client forms tripod position and moves both crutches forward.	
___	___	___	2. Client lifts legs and swings through and ahead of crutches, supporting weight on crutches.	

Excellent	Satisfactory	Needs Practice	

PROCEDURE 34-5
Helping Clients With Crutchwalking (*Continued*)

Goal: To increase client's level of activity after musculo-skeletal injury; to assist client to walk safely with crutches using the least amount of energy.

Comments

Climbing Stairs

1. Use one crutch and the railing. Beginning in tripod position facing stairs, client transfers body weight to crutches and holds onto the railing.
2. Client places unaffected leg on stair.
3. Client transfers body weight to unaffected leg.
4. Client moves crutches and affected leg to stair.
5. Repeat sequence to top of stairs.

Procedure Checklists for Craven and Hirnle's Fundamentals of Nursing: Human Health and Function, 6th edition

Name _____   Date _____

Unit _____   Position _____

Instructor/Evaluator: _____   Position _____

Excellent	Satisfactory	Needs Practice	PROCEDURE 34-6 **Transferring a Client to a Stretcher**	
			Goal: To transfer a client without injuring nurse or client.	**Comments**
___	___	___	1. Identify client. Explain procedure and purpose.	
			2. Place stretcher parallel to bed. Raise bed to same level as stretcher. Lower side rails. Lock wheels.	
___	___	___	3. One or two nurses stand on side of bed without stretcher. Two nurses stand on side of bed with stretcher.	
			4. Loosen draw sheet on both sides of bed.	
___	___	___	5. Nurse on side without stretcher helps client to move toward them onto his or her side. They may use draw sheet to pull client closer.	
___			6. Nurse(s) on stretcher side of bed slide transfer board under draw sheet and under client's buttocks and back.	
___	___	___	7. Place client's arms across his or her chest. Slide client onto transfer board into supine position.	
___	___	___	8. On the count of three, nurse(s) on stretcher side pull the draw sheet toward the stretcher. Nurse on side without transfer board lifts the draw sheet, transferring client's weight to transfer board and pushing client onto stretcher.	
___	___	___	9. Roll client slightly up onto side, and pull transfer sled out from under him or her. Lock up side rails on bed side of stretcher and move stretcher away from bed.	
___	___	___	10. Place sheet over client and lock safety belts across client's chest and waist. Adjust head of stretcher according to client limitations.	

Procedure Checklists for Craven and Hirnle's Fundamentals of Nursing: Human Health and Function, 6th edition

Name _____ Date _____

Unit _____ Position _____

Instructor/Evaluator: _____ Position _____

Excellent	Satisfactory	Needs Practice	PROCEDURE 34-7 **Transferring a Client to a Wheelchair**	Comments
			Goal: To increase mobility status using a wheelchair; to prevent complications of immobility; to increase independence and promote self-esteem.	
___	___	___	1. Identify client and explain procedure.	
___	___	___	2. Position wheelchair at 45-degree angle or parallel to bed. Remove footrest and lock brakes.	
___	___	___	3. Lock bed brakes; lower bed to lowest level, and raise head of bed as far as client can tolerate.	
___	___	___	4. Assist client to side-lying position, facing the side of bed he or she will sit on. Lower side rail and stand near client's hips with foot near head of bed in front of and apart from other foot.	
___	___	___	5. Swing client's legs over side of bed. At the same time, pivot on your back leg to lift client's trunk and shoulders. Keep back straight; avoid twisting. Allow client to independently move to a sitting position if he can tolerate it. Remain close for support.	
___	___	___	6. Stand in front of client, and assess for balance and dizziness. Allow client to dangle legs for a few minutes before continuing.	
___	___	___	7. Help client to don robe and nonskid footwear.	
___	___	___	8. Apply transfer belt. Grip belt to assist with transfer.	
___	___	___	9. Spread your feet apart and flex your hips and knees.	
___	___	___	10. Have client slide buttocks to edge of bed until feet touch floor.	
___	___	___	11. Rock back and forth until client stands on the count of three.	
___	___	___	12. Brace your front knee against client's weak knee as client stands.	
___	___	___	13. Pivot on back foot until client feels wheelchair against back of legs; keep your knee against the client's knee.	
___	___	___	14. Instruct client to place hands on chair armrests for support. Flex your knees and hips while assisting client into chair.	
___	___	___	15. Adjust foot pedal and leg supports.	
___	___	___	16. Assess client's alignment in chair. Provide call light.	

Procedure Checklists for Craven and Hirnle's Fundamentals
of Nursing: Human Health and Function, 6th edition

Name _____   Date _____

Unit _____   Position _____

Instructor/Evaluator: _____   Position _____

Excellent	Satisfactory	Needs Practice	PROCEDURE 34-8 **Procedure for Transferring a Client From Bed to a Chair Using a Hydraulic Lift** **Goal:** To safely transfer a client from a bed to a chair when safe transfer is not possible without using a hydraulic lift.	Comments
___	___	___	1. Identify client and any mobility restrictions. Explain procedure and purpose to client.	
___	___	___	2. Place the fabric sling evenly under the client.	
			3. Position the hydraulic lift so the frame can be centered over the client. Attach the fabric sling to the frame. Note manufacturer's instructions for the specifics of how the sling should be attached to the frame.	
___	___	___	4. Have a nurse on each side of the hydraulic lift. Warn the client that he or she will be lifted from the bed. Support head or heavy casts as needed. Engage the hydraulic system to raise the client from the bed.	
___	___	___	5. Carefully wheel the client in hydraulic lift away from the bed, supporting limbs as needed. Position client over chair and gently lower to chair using the hydraulic mechanism.	
___	___	___	6. The sling remains in place under the client and is reattached to the frame when the client is moved back to bed.	

Procedure Checklists for Craven and Hirnle's Fundamentals of Nursing: Human Health and Function, 6th edition

Name _____   Date _____

Unit _____   Position _____

Instructor/Evaluator: _____   Position _____

Excellent	Satisfactory	Needs Practice	PROCEDURE 35-1 **Monitoring With Pulse Oximetry**	Comments
			Goal: To monitor arterial oxygen saturation (SaO_2) non-invasively; to detect clinical hypoxemia promptly; to assess client's tolerance to tapering of oxygen therapy or activity.	
____	____	____	1. Select appropriate type of sensor. A wide variety of sensors are available in sizes for neonates, infants, children, and adults. In addition, there are clip-on, adhesive, and disposable sensors. To select the appropriate sensor, consider the client's weight, activity level, if infection control is a concern, tape allergies, and anticipated duration of monitoring.	
____	____	____	2. Explain purpose of procedure to client and family.	
____	____	____	3. Instruct client to breathe normally.	
____	____	____	4. Select appropriate site to place sensor. Avoid using lower extremities that may have compromised circulation, or extremities receiving infusions or other invasive monitoring. If client has poor tissue perfusion due to peripheral vascular disease or is receiving vasoconstrictor medications, a nasal sensor or forehead sensor may be considered.	
____	____	____	5. Remove nail polish or acrylic nail from digit to be used.	
____	____	____	6. Attach sensor probe and connect it to the pulse oximeter. Make sure the photosensors are accurately aligned.	
____	____	____	7. Watch for pulse-sensing bar on face of oximeter to fluctuate with each pulsation and reflect pulse strength. Double-check machine pulsations with client's radial or apical pulse.	
____	____	____	8. If continuous pulse oximetry is desired, set the alarm limits on the monitor to reflect the high and low oxygen saturation and pulse rates. Ensure that the alarms are audible before leaving the client. Inspect the sensor site every 4 hours for tissue irritation or pressure from the sensor.	
____	____	____	9. Read saturation on monitor and document as appropriate with all relevant information on client's chart. Report SaO_2 less than 93% to physician.	

Procedure Checklists for Craven and Hirnle's Fundamentals of Nursing: Human Health and Function, 6th edition

Name _____ Date _____

Unit _____ Position _____

Instructor/Evaluator: _____ Position _____

PROCEDURE 35-2
Monitoring Peak Flow

Goal: To measure peak expiratory flow rate (PEFR), which is the point of highest flow during maximal exhalation; to better control asthma by quickly detecting subtle changes in airway diameter so preventive interventions can be instituted; to provide objective data to assess respiratory function.

Excellent	Satisfactory	Needs Practice		Comments
___	___	___	1. Verify the physician order and identify the client.	
___	___	___	2. Explain the purpose of peak flow monitoring to the client and family.	
			3. Place indicator at the base of the numbered scale. Have client stand up.	
___	___	___	4. Tell the client to take a deep breath. Place the meter in his or her mouth. The client should close the lips around the mouthpiece. Remind the client not to put the tongue in the hole.	
___	___	___	5. Tell the client to exhale as fast and as hard as he or she can, keeping a tight fit around the mouthpiece.	
___	___	___	6. Repeat steps 2 through 4 twice more, and record the highest peak flow obtained in the three attempts.	
___	___	___	7. To determine "personal best" when beginning peak flow monitoring, obtain peak flow measurements in the morning and again in the evening over a 2-week period of good asthma control (feel good without any asthma symptoms). The client should take measurements before using bronchodilators.	
___	___	___	8. Healthcare provider will calculate zones based on percentage of personal best (green 80%–100%; yellow 50%–80%; red below 50%) and give instructions for what to do when in each zone.	
___	___	___	9. Encourage client to comply with twice-a-day (morning and evening) peak flow monitoring before bronchodilator therapy and follow healthcare provider's instructions for peak flows in each zone. Follow steps 2 through 5.	

Procedure Checklists for Craven and Hirnle's Fundamentals of Nursing: Human Health and Function, 6th edition

Name _____ Date _____

Unit _____ Position _____

Instructor/Evaluator: _____ Position _____

PROCEDURE 35-3
Teaching Deep-Breathing and Coughing

Excellent	Satisfactory	Needs Practice		Comments

Goal: To facilitate respiratory functioning by increasing lung expansion and preventing alveolar collapse; to encourage expectoration of mucus and secretions that accumulate in the airways after general anesthesia and immobility.

Deep Breathing

1. Assist client to Fowler's or sitting position.
2. Have client place hands palm down, with middle fingers touching, along lower border of rib cage.
3. Ask client to inhale slowly through the nose, feeling middle fingers separate. Hold breath for 2 or 3 seconds.
4. Have client exhale slowly through mouth. Repeat three to five times.

Controlled Coughing

1. If adventitious breath sounds or sputum is present, have client take a deep breath, hold for 3 seconds, and cough deeply two or three times. Stand to the client's side to ensure the cough is not directed at you. Client must cough deeply, not just clear the throat.
2. If the client has an abdominal or chest incision that will cause pain during coughing, instruct the client to hold a pillow firmly over the incision (splinting) when coughing.
3. Instruct, reinforce, and supervise deep-breathing and coughing exercises every 2 to 3 hours postoperatively.
4. Document procedure.

Procedure Checklists for Craven and Hirnle's Fundamentals of Nursing: Human Health and Function, 6th edition

Name _____   Date _____

Unit _____   Position _____

Instructor/Evaluator: _____   Position _____

PROCEDURE 35-4
Promoting Breathing With the Incentive Spirometer

Goal: To provide incentives via visual clues to the client regarding effective deep breathing; to improves pulmonary ventilation and oxygenation, loosens respiratory secretions, and prevents or treats atelectasis by expanding collapsed alveoli.

Excellent	Satisfactory	Needs Practice		Comments
___	___	___	1. Verify the physician order and identify the client.	
___	___	___	2. Wash your hands.	
___	___	___	3. Assist client to high Fowler's or sitting position.	
___	___	___	4. Determine the volume to set incentive spirometry goal based on calculated lung volumes. You may use chart or have respiratory therapy calculated. Set volume indicator. Explain goal to client.	
			5. Instruct client in procedure:	
___	___	___	a. Seal lips tightly around mouthpiece.	
___	___	___	b. Inhale slowly and deeply through mouth. Hold breath for 2 or 3 seconds.	
___	___	___	c. Have client observe his or her progress by watching the balls elevate or lights go on, depending on type of equipment used.	
___	___	___	d. Exhale slowly around mouthpiece and breathe normally for several breaths.	
___	___	___	6. Repeat procedure 5 to 10 times every 1 to 2 hours, per physician's orders.	

Procedure Checklists for Craven and Hirnle's Fundamentals of Nursing: Human Health and Function, 6th edition

Name _____   Date _____

Unit _____   Position _____

Instructor/Evaluator: _____   Position _____

Excellent	Satisfactory	Needs Practice	PROCEDURE 35-5 **Administering Oxygen by Nasal Cannula or Mask**	Comments
			Goal: To deliver low to moderate levels of oxygen to relieve hypoxia.	
___	___	___	1. Review chart for physician's order for oxygen to ensure that it includes method of delivery, flow rate, titration orders; identify client.	
___	___	___	2. Wash your hands.	
___	___	___	3. Identify client and proceed with 5 rights of medication administration. Explain procedure to client. Explain that oxygen will ease dyspnea or discomfort, and inform client concerning safety precautions associated with oxygen use. If the client is using the cannula, encourage him or her to breathe through the nose.	
___	___	___	4. Assist client to semi- or high Fowler's position, if tolerated.	
___	___	___	5. Insert flowmeter into wall outlet. Attach oxygen tubing to nozzle on flowmeter. If using a high O_2 flow, attach humidifier. Attach oxygen tubing to humidifier.	
___	___	___	6. Turn on the oxygen at the prescribed rate. Check that oxygen is flowing through tubing.	
			7. Cannula.	
___	___	___	a. Hold nasal cannula in proper position with prongs curving downward.	
___	___	___	b. Place cannula prongs into nares.	
___	___	___	c. Wrap tubing over and behind ears.	
___	___	___	d. Adjust plastic slide under chin until cannula fits snugly.	
___	___	___	e. Place gauze at ear beneath tubing as necessary.	
___	___	___	f. If prongs dislodge from nares, replace promptly.	
			8. Mask.	
___	___	___	a. Place mask on face, applying from the nose and over the chin.	
___	___	___	b. Adjust the metal rim over the nose and contour the mask to the face.	
___	___	___	c. Adjust elastic band around head so mask fits snugly.	
___	___	___	9. Assess for proper functioning of equipment and observe client's initial response to therapy.	
___	___	___	10. Monitor continuous therapy by assessing for pressure areas on the skin and nares every 2 hours and rechecking flow rate every 4 to 8 hours.	

Procedure Checklists for Craven and Hirnle's Fundamentals
of Nursing: Human Health and Function, 6th edition

Name _____   Date _____

Unit _____   Position _____

Instructor/Evaluator: _____   Position _____

Excellent	Satisfactory	Needs Practice	PROCEDURE 35-6 **Monitoring a Client With a Chest Drainage System** **Goal:** To monitor respiratory status of a patient with a chest tube; to ensure chest drainage system is functioning adequately to promote lung expansion.	Comments
____	____	____	1. Confirm physician's order including amount of suction.	
____	____	____	2. Assist client to semi- or high Fowler's position.	
____	____	____	3. Assess insertion site of chest tube. Note and document amount and color of drainage on dressing around insertion site. Feel insertion site for crepitus—air leaking into the subcutaneous tissue. Document any crepitus found. Reinforce insertion dressing as needed.	
____	____	____	4. Assess status of chest tubing. Be sure tubing remains at the level of the client and no dependent loops are present. Assess that there are no visible clots in the tubing. You may gently "milk" (compress tubing with fingers) the clots to encourage movement into the drainage system, but you never want to strip chest tubing.	
____	____	____	5. Assess the drainage collection chamber. Be sure to keep chest drainage system upright. Assess for amount, color, and character of drainage. Mark the collection chamber to accurately reflect the amount of drainage accumulated during your shift. Note any significant increase in the amount of drainage.	
____	____	____	6. Assess suction chamber. Make sure the water level in the suction chamber is at the prescribed amount of suction and that it is connected to the wall suction that is turned on to continuous suction. Usually the suction is set at 10 to 20 mm Hg.	
____	____	____	7. Assess the system for any air leaks. Check all external connections (i.e., the chest tube's connection to the drainage system, the suction tubing's connection to the drainage system). Examine the water seal chamber as the client breathes normally and as he or she coughs.	
____	____	____	8. Encourage the client to cough, deep breathe, and use an incentive spirometer frequently. Provide analgesics as necessary.	
____	____	____	9. Clamping chest tubes is no longer recommended.	

Excellent	Satisfactory	Needs Practice	PROCEDURE 35-6 **Monitoring a Client With a Chest Drainage System** (*Continued*)	
			Goal: To monitor respiratory status of a patient with a chest tube; to ensure chest drainage system is functioning adequately to promote lung expansion.	**Comments**
____	____	____	10. If the chest tube becomes expelled, do not leave the client. Cover the opening where the chest tube had been inserted with the sterile 4″ × 4″ gauze, and keep direct pressure on the site. Send a colleague to call the physician immediately.	
____	____	____	11. Document chest tube drainage, chest tube patency, presence of an air leak, amount of suction, pain level, dressing status, and respiratory status.	

Procedure Checklists for Craven and Hirnle's Fundamentals
of Nursing: Human Health and Function, 6th edition

Name _____   Date _____

Unit _____   Position _____

Instructor/Evaluator: _____   Position _____

Excellent	Satisfactory	Needs Practice	PROCEDURE 35-7 **Providing Tracheostomy Care** **Goal:** To maintain airway patency by removing mucus and encrusted secretions; to promote cleanliness and prevent infection and skin breakdown at stoma site.	Comments
____	____	____	1. Verify the physician order and identify the client.	
____	____	____	2. Wash your hands and don gloves.	
____	____	____	3. Explain procedure to client. Place the client in semi- to high Fowler's position.	
____	____	____	4. Suction tracheostomy tube. Before discarding gloves, remove soiled tracheostomy dressing and discard with catheter inside glove. *Note:* Follow Procedure 36-8, Suctioning Secretions From Airways. When suctioning through a tracheostomy tube, insert catheter about 10 to 12 cm (in an adult).	
____	____	____	5. Replace oxygen or humidification source and encourage client to deep-breathe as you prepare sterile supplies. Do not snap in place.	
____	____	____	6. Open sterile tracheostomy kit. Pour normal saline into one basin, hydrogen peroxide into the second. Don Sterile gloves. Open several sterile cotton-tipped applicators and one sterile precut tracheostomy dressing and place on sterile field. If kit does not contain tracheostomy ties, cut two 15-inch pieces of twill tape and set aside.	
____	____	____	7. Remove oxygen source. The hand that touches the oxygen source is no longer sterile. *Note:* For tracheostomy tube with inner cannula, complete Steps 7 to 25. For tracheostomy tube without inner cannula or plugged with a button, complete Steps 14 to 25.	
____	____	____	8. Unlock inner cannula by turning counterclockwise. Remove inner cannula.	
____	____	____	9. Place inner cannula in basin with hydrogen peroxide.	
____	____	____	10. Replace oxygen source over or near outer cannula.	
____	____	____	11. Clean lumen and sides of inner cannula using pipe cleaners or sterile brush.	
____	____	____	12. Rinse inner cannula thoroughly by agitating in normal saline for several seconds.	
____	____	____	13. Remove oxygen source and replace inner cannula into outer cannula. "Lock" by turning clockwise until the two blue dots align. Replace oxygen or humidity source.	
____	____	____	14. Remove tracheostomy dressing from under faceplate.	

PROCEDURE 35-7

Providing Tracheostomy Care (*Continued*)

Excellent	Satisfactory	Needs Practice		Comments
			Goal: To maintain airway patency by removing mucus and encrusted secretions; to promote cleanliness and prevent infection and skin breakdown at stoma site.	

____ ____ ____   15. Clean stoma under faceplate with circular motion using hydrogen peroxide-soaked cotton applicators. Clean dried secretions from all exposed outer cannula surfaces.

____ ____ ____   16. Remove foaming secretions using normal saline-soaked, cotton-tipped applicators.

____ ____ ____   17. Pat moist surfaces dry with 4″ × 4″ gauze.

____ ____ ____   18. Place dry, sterile, precut tracheostomy dressing around tracheostomy stoma and under faceplate. Do not use cut 4″ × 4″ gauze.

____ ____ ____   19. If tracheostomy ties are to be changed, have an assistant don a sterile glove and hold the tracheostomy tube in place.

For Tracheostomy Ties, Follow Steps 20-24

____ ____ ____   20. Cut a 12-inch slit approximately 1 inch from one end of both clean tracheostomy ties. This is easily done by folding back on itself 1 inch of the tie and cutting a small slit in the middle.

____ ____ ____   21. Remove and discard soiled tracheostomy ties.

____ ____ ____   22. Thread end of tie through cut slit in tie. Pull tight.

____ ____ ____   23. Repeat Step 21 with the second tie.

____ ____ ____   24. Bring both ties together at one side of the client's neck. Assess that ties are only tight enough to allow one finger between tie and neck. Use two square knots to secure the ties. Trim excess tie length. *Note:* Assess tautness of tracheostomy ties frequently in clients whose neck may swell from trauma or surgery.

For Tracheostomy Collar, Follow Steps 25-27.

____ ____ ____   25. While an assisting nurse holds the faceplate, gently pull the Velcro tab and remove the collar on one side. Insert the new collar into the opening on the faceplate and secure the Velcro tab.

____ ____ ____   26. Hold faceplate in place as the assisting nurse repeats step on the second side.

____ ____ ____   27. Remove the old collar and ensure that the new collar is securely in place.

____ ____ ____   28. Remove gloves and discard disposable equipment. Label with date and time, and store reusable supplies.

____ ____ ____   29. Assist client to comfortable position and offer oral hygiene.

____ ____ ____   30. Wash your hands.

Procedure Checklists for Craven and Hirnle's Fundamentals
of Nursing: Human Health and Function, 6th edition

Name _____   Date _____

Unit _____   Position _____

Instructor/Evaluator: _____   Position _____

Excellent	Satisfactory	Needs Practice	PROCEDURE 35-8 **Suctioning Secretions From Airways**	
			Goal: To remove excess mucous secretions to maintain patent airway; to collect sputum or secretions for diagnostic testing.	**Comments**
____	____	____	1. Verify the physician order and identify the client.	
____	____	____	2. Wash your hands.	
____	____	____	3. Explain procedure and purpose to client.	
____	____	____	4. a. Position the conscious client with an intact gag reflex in a semi-Fowler's position. b. Position the unconscious client in a side-lying position facing you.	
____	____	____	5. Turn on suction device and adjust pressure: infants and children, 50 to 75 mm Hg; adults, 100 to 120 mm Hg.	

____	____	____	6. Open and prepare sterile suction catheter kit.
			  a. Unfold sterile cup, touching only the outside. Place on bedside table.
			  b. Pour sterile saline into cup.	

____	____	____	7. Preoxygenate client with 100% oxygen. Hyperinflate with manual resuscitation bag.	
____	____	____	8. Don sterile gloves. If kit provides only one glove, place on dominant hand.	
____	____	____	9. Pick up catheter with dominant hand. Pick up connecting tubing with nondominant hand. The nondominant hand is now considered clean rather than sterile. Attach catheter to tubing without contaminating sterile hand.	
____	____	____	10. Place catheter end into cup of saline. Test functioning of equipment by applying thumb from nondominant hand over open port to create suction.	
____	____	____	11. Insert catheter into trachea through nostril, nasal trumpet, or artificial airway during inspiration.	
____	____	____	12. Advance catheter until you feel resistance. Retract catheter 1 cm before applying suction. *Note:* Client usually will cough when catheter enters trachea.	
____	____	____	13. Apply suction by placing thumb of nondominant hand over open port. Rotate the catheter with your dominant hand as you withdraw the catheter. This should take 5 to 10 seconds	
____	____	____	14. Hyperoxygenate and hyperinflate using manual resuscitation bag for a full minute between subsequent suction passes. Encourage deep breathing.	

PROCEDURE 35-8
Suctioning Secretions From Airways (*Continued*)

Goal: To remove excess mucous secretions to maintain patent airway; to collect sputum or secretions for diagnostic testing.

Excellent	Satisfactory	Needs Practice		Comments
____	____	____	15. Rinse catheter thoroughly with saline.	
____	____	____	16. Repeat Steps 10 to 14 until airway is clear, limiting each suctioning to three passes.	
____	____	____	17. Without applying suction, insert the catheter gently along one side of the mouth. Advance to the oropharynx.	
____	____	____	18. Apply suction for 5 to 10 seconds as you rotate and withdraw catheter.	
____	____	____	19. Allow 1 to 2 minutes between passes for the client to ventilate. Encourage deep breathing. Replace oxygen if applicable.	
____	____	____	20. Repeat Steps 16 and 17 as necessary to clear oropharynx.	
____	____	____	21. Rinse catheter and tubing by suctioning saline through.	
____	____	____	22. Remove gloves by holding catheter with dominant hand and pulling glove off inside-out. Catheter will remain coiled inside the glove. Pull other glove off inside-out. Dispose of in trash receptacle.	
____	____	____	23. Turn off suction device.	
____	____	____	24. Assist client to comfortable position. Offer assistance with oral and nasal hygiene. Replace oxygen device if used.	
____	____	____	25. Dispose of disposable supplies.	
____	____	____	26. Wash your hands.	
____	____	____	27. Ensure that sterile suction kit is available at head of bed.	

Procedure Checklists for Craven and Hirnle's Fundamentals of Nursing: Human Health and Function, 6th edition

Name _____   Date _____

Unit _____   Position _____

Instructor/Evaluator: _____   Position _____

Excellent	Satisfactory	Needs Practice	PROCEDURE 35-9 **Managing an Obstructed Airway (Heimlich Maneuver)**	Comments
			Goal: To remove a foreign body from obstructing the airway to prevent anoxia and cardiopulmonary arrest.	
			Conscious Child or Adult (Heimlich Maneuver)	
____	____	____	1. The client will be standing or sitting.	
____	____	____	2. Stand behind the client.	
____	____	____	3. Wrap your arms around client's waist.	
____	____	____	4. Make a fist with one hand. Place thumb side of fist against client's abdomen, above the navel but below the xiphoid process.	
____	____	____	5. Grasp fist with other hand.	
____	____	____	6. Press fist into abdomen with a quick upward thrust.	
____	____	____	7. Repeat distinct separate thrusts until the client expels the foreign body or becomes unconscious.	
			Unconscious Client (Heimlich Maneuver, Abdominal Thrust)	
____	____	____	1. Client will be lying on the ground.	
____	____	____	2. Turn client on back and call for help. Activate emergency response system.	
____	____	____	3. Finger sweep.	
____	____	____	a. Use tongue–jaw lift to open mouth.	
____	____	____	b. Insert index finger inside cheek and sweep to base of tongue if an object is visible. Use a hooking motion if possible to dislodge and remove the foreign body. *Note:* Avoid finger sweeps in infants and children because you can easily push the foreign body further into the airway. Remove only if clearly visible and easy to reach.	
____	____	____	c. If there is no effective breathing, attempt to provide 2 rescue breaths. If unsuccessful, reposition and try to ventilate again.	
____	____	____	4. Straddle client's thighs or kneel to the side of thighs.	
____	____	____	5. Place heel of one hand on epigastric area, midline above the navel but below the xiphoid process.	
____	____	____	6. Place second hand on top of first hand.	
____	____	____	7. Press heel of hand into abdomen with a quick upward thrust. *Note:* Be careful to thrust in the midline to prevent injury to the liver or spleen.	

Excellent	Satisfactory	Needs Practice	PROCEDURE 35-9 **Managing an Obstructed Airway (Heimlich Maneuver)** (*Continued*)	
			Goal: To remove a foreign body from obstructing the airway to prevent anoxia and cardiopulmonary arrest.	**Comments**
____	____	____	8. Repeat abdominal thrusts 5 times.	
____	____	____	9. If airway is still obstructed, attempt to ventilate using mouth-to-mouth respiration and head tilt/chin lift.	
____	____	____	10. Repeat Steps 5 through 8 until successful.	
			Children Younger Than 1 Year of Age (Back Blows and Chest Thrusts)	
____	____	____	1. Straddle infant over your arm with head lower than trunk.	
____	____	____	2. Support head by holding jaw firmly in your hand.	
____	____	____	3. Rest your forearm on your thigh and deliver five back blows with the heel of your hand between the infant's scapula.	
____	____	____	4. Place free hand on infant's back and support neck while turning to supine position.	
____	____	____	5. Place two fingers over sternum in same location as for external chest compression (one fingerwidth below nipple line).	
____	____	____	6. Administer five chest thrusts.	
____	____	____	7. Repeat Steps 1 through 6 until airway is not obstructed.	
			Children Older Than 1 Year of Age	
____	____	____	1. Perform Heimlich maneuver with child standing, sitting, or lying as for adult, but more gently.	
____	____	____	2. You may need to kneel behind child or have child stand on a table.	
____	____	____	3. Prevent foreign body airway obstruction in infants and children by teaching parents or caregivers to:	
____	____	____	a. Restrict children from walking, running, or playing with food or foreign objects in their mouths.	
____	____	____	b. Keep small objects (e.g., marbles, beads, beans, thumb tacks) away from children younger than 3 years of age.	
____	____	____	c. Avoid feeding popcorn and peanuts to children younger than 3 years of age, and cut other foods into small pieces.	
____	____	____	4. Instruct parents and caregivers in the management of foreign body airway obstruction.	

Excellent	Satisfactory	Needs Practice	PROCEDURE 35-9 **Managing an Obstructed Airway (Heimlich Maneuver)** (***Continued***)	
			Goal: To remove a foreign body from obstructing the airway to prevent anoxia and cardiopulmonary arrest.	**Comments**

Pregnant Women or Very Obese Adults (Chest Thrusts)

___	___	___	1. Stand behind client.
___	___	___	2. Bring your arms under client's armpits and around chest.
___	___	___	3. Make a fist and place thumb side against middle of sternum.
___	___	___	4. Grasp fist with other hand and deliver a quick backward thrust.
___	___	___	5. Repeat thrusts until airway is cleared.
			6. Chest thrusts may be performed with client supine and hands positioned with heel over lower half of sternum (as for cardiac compression). Administer separate downward thrusts until airway is clear

*Procedure Checklists for Craven and Hirnle's Fundamentals
of Nursing: Human Health and Function,* 6th edition

Name _____   Date _____

Unit _____   Position _____

Instructor/Evaluator: _____   Position _____

Excellent	Satisfactory	Needs Practice	PROCEDURE 36-1 **Applying Antiembolic Stockings** **Goal:** To promote supplementing the action of muscle contraction by venous return from the legs; to prevent deep vein thrombosis in the immobile client.	Comments
____	____	____	1. Position client in supine position for a half-hour before applying stockings.	
____	____	____	2. Provide for the client's privacy and explain the purpose of the antiembolic stockings.	
____	____	____	3. Measure for proper fit before first application. Measure length (heel to groin) and width (calf and thigh) and compare to manufacturer's printed material to ensure proper fit.	
____	____	____	4. Make sure legs are dry or apply a light dusting of powder.	
____	____	____	5. Turn the stocking inside out, tucking the foot inside.	
____	____	____	6. Ease foot section over the client's toe and heel, adjusting as necessary for proper smooth fit.	
____	____	____	7. Gently pull the stocking over the leg, removing all wrinkles.	
____	____	____	8. Assess toes for circulation and warmth. Check area at top of stocking for binding.	
____	____	____	9. Antiembolic stockings should be removed at least twice daily.	

Procedure Checklists for Craven and Hirnle's Fundamentals
of Nursing: Human Health and Function, 6th edition

Name _____   Date _____

Unit _____   Position _____

Instructor/Evaluator: _____   Position _____

Excellent	Satisfactory	Needs Practice	PROCEDURE 36-2 **Applying a Sequential Compression Device (SCD)** **Goal:** To promote venous return from legs to decrease the risk of deep vein thrombosis and pulmonary embolism in clients with reduced mobility.	Comments
____	____	____	1. Measure leg to ensure proper sleeve sizing. *Note:* Knee length—one size fits all; thigh length—measure length of leg from ankle to popliteal fossa. Measure circumference of thigh at the gluteal fold. Use the correct sleeve size, as follows: extra small (circumference, 22 inches; length, 16 inches); regular (circumference, 29 inches; length, 16 inches); extra large (circumference, 35 inches; length, 16 inches).	
____	____	____	2. Apply antiembolism stockings. Ensure that there are no wrinkles or folds (see Procedure 36-1). *Note:* Stockinette or Ace wraps are recommended options if client cannot be fitted with antiembolism stockings.	
____	____	____	3. Place client in supine position.	
____	____	____	4. Place a plastic sleeve under each leg so that the opening is at the knee. If only one sleeve is required, leave the other sleeve in package and connect to control unit.	
____	____	____	5. Fold the outer section of the sleeve over the inner portion and secure with Velcro tabs. Check sleeve fit. Two fingers should fit between the sleeve and leg.	
____	____	____	6. Connect tubing to control unit. The premarked arrows on the tubing from the sleeve and from the controller must be aligned to make adequate connection. Turn machine on.	
____	____	____	7. Adjust control unit settings as necessary. Unit control is preset with sleeve cooling in "off" position and audible alarm in "on" position. Sleeve cooling should be in "on" position at all times except during surgery. Ankle pressure should be set at 35–55 mm Hg.	
____	____	____	8. Recheck control unit settings whenever unit has been turned off.	
____	____	____	9. Respond to and promptly correct all "fault" indicator alarms. *Note:* The control unit will sense and indicate four pressure "fault" conditions: (a) pressure failed to drop to zero during the cycle;	

PROCEDURE 36-2
Applying a Sequential Compression Device (SCD) (*Continued*)

Goal: To promote venous return from legs to decrease the risk of deep vein thrombosis and pulmonary embolism in clients with reduced mobility.

Excellent	Satisfactory	Needs Practice		Comments
			(b) the ankle pressure failed to reach 20 mm Hg for five consecutive cycles; (c) the ankle pressure exceeded 90 mm Hg; (d) internal diagnostics error has occurred.	
___	___	___	10. Document time and date of application. If SCD is applied to only one leg, document reason.	
___	___	___	11. Assess and document skin integrity every 8 hours.	
___	___	___	12. Remove sleeves and notify physician if client experiences tingling, numbness, or leg pain.	

Procedure Checklists for Craven and Hirnle's Fundamentals
of Nursing: Human Health and Function, 6th edition

Name _____   Date _____

Unit _____   Position _____

Instructor/Evaluator: _____   Position _____

Excellent	Satisfactory	Needs Practice	PROCEDURE 38-1 **Measuring Blood Glucose by Skin Puncture** **Goal:** To monitor blood glucose levels for clients who are at risk for hypoglycemia or hyperglycemia; to monitor the effectiveness of insulin administration.	Comments
____	____	____	1. Have the client wash hands with soap and warm water.	
____	____	____	2. Position client comfortably.	
____	____	____	3. Remove the test strip from the container and handle according to the manufacturer's instructions.	
____	____	____	4. Place the test strip with test pad up on a dry surface.	
____	____	____	5. Don gloves.	
____	____	____	6. Choose the finger to be punctured, massage gently, and hold in a dependent position.	
____	____	____	7. Wipe the puncture site with alcohol. Allow the site to dry completely.	
____	____	____	8. Remove the cover of the lancet or autolet. Place the autolet against the side of the finger and push the release button. If using a lancet, hold it perpendicular to the site and pierce the site quickly.	
____	____	____	9. Squeeze the finger gently or milk the skin toward the puncture site to obtain a large drop of blood. Hold the test strip next to the drop of blood and allow the blood to cover the test pad completely. Do not smear the blood. In some meters, bring the finger to the test site on the meter and allow blood to drop and wick along the test strip, covering the test strip area.	
____	____	____	10. Start the timing (usually less than 60 seconds) using the glucose meter, or use a watch if the meter is not available.	
____	____	____	11. Place the test strip into the glucose meter. After the recommended period, read the results. For meters on which blood is placed directly, read the results at the designated time. If a glucose meter is not available, compare the color of the test pad with the color strip on the side of the reagent strip container.	
____	____	____	12. Turn off the glucose meter. Dispose of used equipment in the appropriate manner.	
____	____	____	13. Share test results with client and record obtained values in the client's chart.	

Procedure Checklists for Craven and Hirnle's Fundamentals of Nursing: Human Health and Function, 6th edition

Name _____ Date _____

Unit _____ Position _____

Instructor/Evaluator: _____ Position _____

Excellent	Satisfactory	Needs Practice	PROCEDURE 38-2 **Assisting an Adult With Feeding**	Comments
			Goal: To maintain nutritional status; to provide a time for socialization.	
___	___	___	1. Prepare client's environment for meal:	
___	___	___	a. Remove urinals, bedpans, dressings, trash.	
___	___	___	b. Ventilate or aerate room for unpleasant odors.	
___	___	___	c. Clean overbed table.	
___	___	___	2. Prepare client for meal:	
___	___	___	a. Help client urinate or defecate.	
___	___	___	b. Help client wash face and hands.	
___	___	___	c. Assist with oral hygiene.	
___	___	___	d. Help client apply dentures, glasses, or special appliances.	
___	___	___	e. Assist to upright position in bed or chair.	
___	___	___	3. Wash your hands before touching meal tray.	
___	___	___	4. Check client's tray against diet order and with client's identification.	
___	___	___	5. Place tray on overbed table and move in front of client.	
___	___	___	6. Place a napkin or towel under client's chin, and cover clothing. Prepare tray. Open cartons, remove lids, season food, cut food into bite-size pieces.	
___	___	___	7. If client can feed self, you may leave at this point. Return after 10 to 15 minutes to determine whether client is tolerating diet. Do not leave clients with overly hot liquids or food unless they are fully independent with feeding.	
___	___	___	8. Assist clients who cannot feed themselves. If client can sit in a chair but needs help to eat, sit in chair facing client. If client must remain in bed, sit in chair (depending on chair height) or stand to feed client.	
___	___	___	9. Allow client to choose the order he or she would like to eat. If client is visually impaired, identify the food on the tray.	
___	___	___	10. Warn client if food is hot or cold. Allow enough time between bites for adequate chewing and swallowing.	
___	___	___	11. Offer liquids as requested or between bites. Use a straw or special drinking cup if available.	
___	___	___	12. Provide conversation during meal. Choose topic of interest to client. Reorient to current events, or use	

PROCEDURE 38-2
Assisting an Adult With Feeding (*Continued*)

Excellent	Satisfactory	Needs Practice	**Goal:** To maintain nutritional status; to provide a time for socialization.	Comments
			meal as an opportunity to educate on nutrition or discharge plans. However, do not talk to clients who are relearning swallowing techniques; they need to concentrate.	
___	___	___	13. Remove and dispose of tray. Help client wash hands and face and perform oral hygiene after meal.	
___	___	___	14. Assist to comfortable position, and allow rest period. Note: If client is at risk for aspiration, leave head of bed elevated for 30 minutes after eating.	
___	___	___	15. Record fluids and amount of meal consumed, if ordered.	
___	___	___	16. Wash your hands.	

Procedure Checklists for Craven and Hirnle's Fundamentals of Nursing: Human Health and Function, 6th edition

Name _____   Date _____

Unit _____   Position _____

Instructor/Evaluator: _____   Position _____

PROCEDURE 38-3
Administering Specialized Nutritional Support Via Small-Bore Nasogastric, Gastrostomy, or Jejunostomy Tube

Goal: To provide enteral nutrition for clients who cannot swallow or who have an esophageal obstruction; to provide nutrition to comatose or semiconscious clients; to provide additional nutrients for clients who cannot orally consume adequate calories.

Excellent	Satisfactory	Needs Practice		Comments
____	____	____	1. Wash your hands and don gloves.	
____	____	____	2. Close room door or curtains around bed.	
____	____	____	3. Explain procedure to client.	
____	____	____	4. Help client to Fowler's position by elevating head of bed at least 30 to 45 degrees or assisting to a chair. If an upright position is contraindicated, help client to a right side-lying position with head elevated 30 degrees.	
____	____	____	5. Confirm placement of tube. Attach 60-mL irrigation syringe to tube and inject 10 to 20 mL of air while auscultating with the stethoscope:	
____	____	____	• Stomach: Auscultation heard best in the midline and left upper quadrant.	
____	____	____	• Duodenum: Auscultation heard best over right upper quadrant and radiates to the left upper quadrant.	
____	____	____	• Distal duodenum/proximal jejunum: Air is heard loudest in the left flank area.	
____	____	____	6. Check gastric residual volumes (GRVs).	
____	____	____	a. If GRVs are requested, note amount aspirated in documentation. Notify provider if GRV exceeds 400 to 500 mL.	
____	____	____	b. Replace all gastric contents after residual check.	
____	____	____	7. Prepare correct amount and strength of formula. Formula should be room temperature. Proceed to Step 8 below for bolus or intermittent or continuous feeding.	

Bolus or Intermittent Feeding

Excellent	Satisfactory	Needs Practice		Comments
____	____	____	8. Remove plunger from irrigation syringe. Clamp gastric tubing and attach syringe or feeding bag. If using a feeding bag, prime the tubing and attach feeding bag and tubing to the client's feeding tube.	
____	____	____	9. Fill syringe or feeding bag with formula. Allow feeding to flow in slowly (10–15 minutes). If using	

PROCEDURE 38-3

Administering Specialized Nutritional Support Via Small-Bore Nasogastric, Gastrostomy, or Jejunostomy Tube (*Continued*)

Excellent	Satisfactory	Needs Practice	**Goal:** To provide enteral nutrition for clients who cannot swallow or who have an esophageal obstruction; to provide nutrition to comatose or semiconscious clients; to provide additional nutrients for clients who cannot orally consume adequate calories.	**Comments**
			syringe, raise or lower syringe to adjust flow rate by gravity. Refill syringe as needed without disconnecting, avoiding air spaces in tubing. If a feeding bag is used, hang bag on IV pole, and adjust flow rate with clamp on tubing.	
___	___	___	10. Clamp tubing just as feeding is completing. Rinse tube with 30 to 60 mL warm tap water. Do not allow air to enter tubing.	
___	___	___	11. Clamp gastric tube, and disconnect from syringe or feeding bag.	
___	___	___	12. Have client remain in Fowler's or elevated side-lying position for 30 to 60 minutes after feeding.	
___	___	___	13. Wash any reusable equipment with soap and water. Change equipment every 24 hours or according to agency policy.	
___	___	___	14. Wash hands.	
			15. Document appropriately.	
			Continuous Feeding	
___	___	___	8. Connect feeding bag and tubing to client's feeding tube.	
___	___	___	9. Pour in desired amount of formula. *Note:* Usually hang amount of formula to infuse in 3 hours; check agency policy. Place label on bag with client's name, date, and time feeding was initiated.	
___	___	___	10. Hang feeding bag on IV pole. Allow formula to flow through bag.	
___	___	___	11. Connect tubing to infusion pump and set rate.	
___	___	___	12. Clients receiving continuous feedings should have gastric residuals checked every 4 to 6 hours, according to agency policy. Then flush the tubing with 30 to 60 mL of warm water.	
___	___	___	13. Have client remain in Fowler's or in slightly elevated side-lying position.	
___	___	___	14. Wash any reusable equipment with soap and water. Change equipment every 24 hours or according to agency policy.	
___	___	___	15. Wash hands.	
___	___	___	16. Document appropriately.	

Procedure Checklists for Craven and Hirnle's Fundamentals
of Nursing: Human Health and Function, 6th edition

Name _____   Date _____

Unit _____   Position _____

Instructor/Evaluator: _____   Position _____

PROCEDURE 39-1
Changing a Dry Sterile Dressing

Goal: To protect wound from trauma and external contamination; to provide opportunity to assess the wound; to provide an absorbent covering over the wound.

Columns: Excellent | Satisfactory | Needs Practice | | Comments

1. Close client's door or curtains around bed. Explain procedure to client.
2. Position client comfortably. Expose only wound area.
3. Wash your hands.
4. Ensure that an appropriate waste receptacle is within easy reach of dressing table.
5. Put on clean disposable gloves.
6. Remove dressing from wound, and discard into appropriate waste container. *Note:* If dressing adheres to wound, pour a small amount of sterile saline on the wound to loosen the dressing and prevent disruption of healing tissue.
7. Dispose of gloves. Wash your hands.
8. Set up sterile supplies.
   a. Open sterile drape, and hold it by the edges.
   b. Place it on a clean, flat surface without contaminating the center of the drape.
   c. Open dressing package (or packages) by peeling paper down to expose dressing. Let it fall onto the sterile field.
   d. Open cleansing solution container, and pour solution into sterile cup.
   e. Open any supplies for wound irrigation and set materials at the side of the sterile field.
9. Don sterile gloves. Grasp applicators at non-absorbent end and dip them into the cleansing solution.
10. Clean drainage from the wound's center outward, using each applicator only once and discarding without placing the applicator back into the cleansing solution.
11. Dry the surrounding skin gently with gauze.
12. Inspect the wound for bleeding, inflammation, drainage, and healing. Note any areas of dehiscence (opening or gaping of wound edges).
13. Apply sterile dressings one at a time over the wound.
14. Wash your hands.
15. Document procedure and observations.

*Procedure Checklists for Craven and Hirnle's Fundamentals
of Nursing: Human Health and Function,* 6th edition

Name _____ Date _____

Unit _____ Position _____

Instructor/Evaluator: _____ Position _____

Excellent	Satisfactory	Needs Practice	PROCEDURE 39-2 **Applying a Saline-Moistened Dressing**	Comments
			Goal: To promote moist wound healing; to protect the wound from contamination and mechanical trauma.	
____	____	____	1. Prepare client and remove dressing according to Steps 1 through 5 of Procedure 39-1. *Note:* Forceps may be used to remove a soiled dressing. If dressing adheres to underlying tissues, moisten with saline to loosen. Gently remove the dressing while assessing client's discomfort level.	
____	____	____	2. Observe dressings for amount and characteristics of drainage. Note odor and color.	
____	____	____	3. Observe wound for eschar (thick layer of dead cells and dried plasma), granulation tissue (reddish capillary loops that bleed easily), or epithelial skin buds. Measure and record wound depth, diameter, and length.	
____	____	____	4. Prepare sterile supplies. Open sterile instruments, sterile basin, solution, and dressings. Pour ordered solution into sterile basin.	
____	____	____	5. Don sterile gloves.	
____	____	____	6. Using sterile forceps, withdraw fine-mesh gauze to appropriate length and cut with sterile scissors. Place fine-mesh gauze into basin to saturate.	
____	____	____	7. Cleanse or irrigate wound as prescribed or with normal saline, moving from least to most contaminated areas.	
____	____	____	8. Squeeze excess fluid from gauze dressing. Unfold and fluff out the dressing.	
____	____	____	a. Gently pack moistened gauze into the wound.	
____	____	____	b. If wound is deep, use forceps or cotton-tipped applicators to press gauze into all wound surfaces.	
____	____	____	9. Apply several dry, sterile 4 × 4 pads over the wet gauze.	
____	____	____	10. Place ABD pad over dry 4 × 4 pads, if necessary.	
____	____	____	11. Dispose of sterile gloves.	
____	____	____	12. Secure dressings with tape, Kerlix gauze (for circumferential dressings), or Montgomery ties.	
____	____	____	13. Assist client to a comfortable position.	
____	____	____	14. Wash your hands.	
____	____	____	15. Document procedure and observations.	

Procedure Checklists for Craven and Hirnle's Fundamentals of Nursing: Human Health and Function, 6th edition

Name _____ Date _____

Unit _____ Position _____

Instructor/Evaluator: _____ Position _____

Excellent	Satisfactory	Needs Practice	PROCEDURE 39-3 **Irrigating a Wound**	Comments
			Goal: To cleanse the wound by removing debris and exudate; to instill medication into the wound (if ordered); to promote wound healing.	
___	___	___	1. Close door or curtains around bed. Explain procedure to client.	
___	___	___	2. Position client comfortably to allow irrigating solution to flow by gravity across the wound and into a collection basin.	
___	___	___	3. Expose only the wound area. Place waterproof pad under client.	
___	___	___	4. Wash your hands.	
___	___	___	5. Don mask, goggles, and gown if needed.	
___	___	___	6. Remove dressing and inspect wound. See Steps 1 through 4 of Procedure 39-2.	
___	___	___	7. Pour warmed irrigating solution into sterile irrigation container.	
___	___	___	8. Open irrigating syringe and place into container with solution.	
___	___	___	9. Place a sterile basin at distal end of wound.	
___	___	___	10. Don sterile gloves.	
___	___	___	11. Fill irrigating syringe with solution. Holding syringe tip about 1 inch above the wound, gently flush all wound areas. Continue flushing until solution draining into basin is clear.	
___	___	___	12. If wound is deep, attach a latex or silicone catheter to filled syringe with irrigating solution. Gently insert catheter into wound and flush until returning solution is clear. When refilling irrigation syringe with solution, disconnect catheter, fill syringe, and reconnect catheter (doing so prevents contaminating the basin of solution with microorganisms from the catheter).	
___	___	___	13. Dry surrounding skin thoroughly.	
___	___	___	14. Apply sterile dressing.	
___	___	___	15. Remove and discard gloves.	
___	___	___	16. Secure dressing with tape or Montgomery straps.	
___	___	___	17. Assist client to a comfortable position.	
___	___	___	18. Dispose of equipment. *Note:* Retain remaining bottle of sterile solution for future irrigations. Mark date and time of opening on bottle for reference. Dispose according to agency policy.	
___	___	___	19. Wash your hands.	
___	___	___	20. Document procedure and observations.	

Procedure Checklists for Craven and Hirnle's Fundamentals of Nursing: Human Health and Function, 6th edition

Name _____ Date _____

Unit _____ Position _____

Instructor/Evaluator: _____ Position _____

Excellent	Satisfactory	Needs Practice	PROCEDURE 39-4 **Maintaining a Portable Wound Suction**	
			Goal: To facilitate healing by removing drainage from the incisional area where granulation tissue is forming.	**Comments**
____	____	____	1. Explain procedure; assist client to a comfortable position; pull curtains or close door.	
____	____	____	2. Wash your hands. Don clean disposable gloves.	
____	____	____	3. Expose wound suction tubing and container while keeping client draped.	
____	____	____	4. Examine tubing and container for patency and suction seal. *Note:* If the system's seal is broken, the Hemovac reservoir will be expanded and not compressed.	
			5. Open the drainage plug.	
____	____	____	6. Pour drainage into a calibrated receptacle without contaminating the drainage spout. Use an antiseptic swab to clean the drainage spout.	
____	____	____	7. Reestablish suction. With drainage plug open, compress the unit and reinsert drainage plug.	
____	____	____	8. Remove and discard gloves.	
____	____	____	9. Return client to a comfortable position.	
____	____	____	10. Measure drainage and record amount, color, and any other pertinent information.	

Procedure Checklists for Craven and Hirnle's Fundamentals
of Nursing: Human Health and Function, 6th edition

Name _____   Date _____

Unit _____   Position _____

Instructor/Evaluator: _____   Position _____

Excellent	Satisfactory	Needs Practice	PROCEDURE 39-5 **Application of Heat**	Comments
			Goal: To promote warm, moist wound healing; to increase blood flow, resolve inflammation, improve healing of soft tissues; to relieve muscular pain and stiffness.	
			Commercial Heat Pack (Variations Depending on Source of Thermotherapy)	
____	____	____	1. Perform hand hygiene, identify the client, and explain the procedure.	
____	____	____	2. Remove appropriate-size pack from wrapping paper.	
____	____	____	3. Note the directions for squeezing and rupturing a small vessel that releases the chemical into the larger bag.	
____	____	____	4. Gently mix the bag, checking for leaks.	
____	____	____	5. Apply the pack, checking back in 3 to 5 minutes to inspect the client's skin for erythema.	
____	____	____	6. Remove pack when stated by the physician's order or when it is no longer hot.	
____	____	____	7. Dispose of the heat pack. Do not reuse it.	
			Warm Moist Compresses to an Open Wound	
____	____	____	1. Prepare the client and the wound area as described in Procedure 39-1.	
			2. If dressings are to be soaked in solution prior to placing them over wound, use sterile technique to add the appropriate number of dressings to the sterile solution in the sterile basin.	
____	____	____	3. Wring out dressings prior to applying to wound.	
____	____	____	4. Loosely apply moist sterile dressing.	
			5. Cover the moist dressings with dry dressings or an ABD pad and secure the dressings using tape, Montgomery straps, or towels.	
____	____	____	6. Apply aquathermia unit. If an aquathermia pad is not used to maintain a sustained temperature, the dressings will need to be checked more frequently and changed as needed to meet the requirements of the dressing order.	
			Aquathermia Pad	
____	____	____	1. Check equipment: make sure connections are secure and cords are not frayed.	

PROCEDURE 39-5
Application of Heat (*Continued*)

Excellent	Satisfactory	Needs Practice		Comments
			Goal: To promote warm, moist wound healing; to increase blood flow, resolve inflammation, improve healing of soft tissues; to relieve muscular pain and stiffness.	
——	——	——	2. Turn pump on and set the temperature with the pump key.	
——	——	——	3. Apply the pad with coiled surfaces next to the area to be treated or on the warm moist dressing.	
——	——	——	4. Secure with tape, if needed.	
——	——	——	5. Check the client's skin and area of treatment every 5 minutes for the first 20 minutes to be sure the temperature is well tolerated.	
——	——	——	6. Check water level on aquathermia unit to make sure it is at the appropriate level.	

Procedure Checklists for Craven and Hirnle's Fundamentals of Nursing: Human Health and Function, 6th edition

Name _____ Date _____

Unit _____ Position _____

Instructor/Evaluator: _____ Position _____

Excellent	Satisfactory	Needs Practice	PROCEDURE 40-1 **Obtaining a Wound Culture**	Comments
			Goal: To identify organisms colonized within a wound so that antibiotics sensitive to the microorganisms can be prescribed, as needed.	
____	____	____	1. Identify client using two separate identifiers (e.g., name, medical record number, or birthdate) and verify order for culture noting site and type of culture. Label the specimen container and make sure the information includes the client's name, medical record number, date and time specimen is obtained, and site of the culture.	
____	____	____	2. Wash hands and apply disposable gloves.	
____	____	____	3. Remove soiled dressing. Observe drainage for amount, odor, and color.	
____	____	____	4. Clear and remove exudate from around wound and cleanse with normal saline.	
			Obtaining Aerobic Culture	
____	____	____	1. Perform Steps 1 to 4 above.	
____	____	____	2. Using sterile swab from culture tube, insert swab deep into area of active drainage. Rotate swab to absorb as much drainage as possible.	
____	____	____	3. Insert swab into culture tube, taking care not to touch the top or outside of the tube.	
____	____	____	4. Crush ampule of medium and close container securely.	
____	____	____	5. Continue with Step 4 below.	
			Obtaining Anaerobic Culture	
____	____	____	1. Perform Steps 1 to 4 at beginning of procedure.	
____	____	____	2. Using sterile swab from special anaerobic culture tube, insert swab deeply into draining body cavity.	
____	____	____	3. a. Rotate swab gently and remove. Quickly place swab into inner tube of collection container.	
____	____	____	b. *Alternative method:* Insert tip of syringe with needle removed into wound and aspirate 1 to 5 mL of exudate. Attach 21-gauge needle to syringe, expel all air, and inject exudate into inner tube of the culture container.	
____	____	____	4. Send specimens in the pre-labeled containers with appropriate requisition immediately to the laboratory.	

PROCEDURE 40-1
Obtaining a Wound Culture (*Continued*)

Excellent	Satisfactory	Needs Practice	**Goal:** To identify organisms colonized within a wound so that antibiotics sensitive to the microorganisms can be prescribed, as needed.	**Comments**
			Some agencies require that specimens be transported in clean plastic bags to further prevent transfer of microorganisms.	
____	____	____	5. Clean and apply sterile dressings to the wound, as ordered.	
____	____	____	6. Remove and discard gloves. Wash hands.	
____	____	____	7. Assist client to comfortable position.	
____	____	____	8. Document all relevant information on the client's chart. Include the location the specimen was taken from, and the date and time. Record the wound's appearance, and the color, odor, amount, and consistency of drainage. Record how the client tolerated the procedure and any discomfort that he or she experienced.	

Procedure Checklists for Craven and Hirnle's Fundamentals of Nursing: Human Health and Function, 6th edition

Name _____ Date _____

Unit _____ Position _____

Instructor/Evaluator: _____ Position _____

Excellent	Satisfactory	Needs Practice	PROCEDURE 41-1 **Collecting Urine Specimens**	Comments
			Goal: To obtain a noncontaminated urine specimen for routine analysis or culture and sensitivity.	
			Collecting Sterile Specimen from an Indwelling Catheter	
___	___	___	1. Confirm the physician's order and verify the client using two separate identifiers (name and medical record or birth date).	
___	___	___	2. Explain procedure to client.	
___	___	___	3. Wash hands. Put on disposable gloves.	
___	___	___	4. Close curtains around bed and close door to room if possible. Position client so that catheter is accessible.	
___	___	___	5. Drain urine from tubing into collection bag. Allow fresh urine to collect in tubing by clamping or bending tubing (2 mL of urine is sufficient for a culture and sensitivity specimen, 30 mL for urinalysis).	
___	___	___	6. Cleanse the aspiration port of the drainage tubing with alcohol or antimicrobial swab.	
___	___	___	7. Insert syringe into aspiration port. Draw urine sample into syringe by gentle aspiration. Remove syringe from port and unclamp the drainage tubing.	
___	___	___	8. Transfer urine from syringe into a sterile specimen container.	
___	___	___	9. Identify the client with at least two identifiers (name, medical record number, birth date) and match this information to the label on the container. Note date and time on laboratory requisition form. Place in plastic biohazard bag for delivery to the laboratory.	
___	___	___	10. Send specimen to laboratory within 15 minutes or place in specimen refrigerator. If specimen is for microbiology testing, it must be sent immediately and not refrigerated.	
___	___	___	11. Dispose of all contaminated supplies. Wash hands.	
___	___	___	12. Document procedure and observations.	
			Self-Collecting Midstream Urine Specimen for a Woman	
___	___	___	1. Confirm the order and identify the client using two separate identifiers.	

PROCEDURE 41-1
Collecting Urine Specimens (*Continued*)

Goal: To obtain a noncontaminated urine specimen for routine analysis or culture and sensitivity.

Excellent	Satisfactory	Needs Practice		Comments
____	____	____	2. Give the client the following instructions on how to cleanse urinary meatus and obtain a urine specimen: a. Wash hands.	
____	____	____	b. Separate labia minora and cleanse perineum with commercially prepared aseptic swabs, starting in front of the urethral meatus and moving swab toward the rectum.	
____	____	____	c. Repeat this cleansing process three times with different cotton balls or swabs.	
____	____	____	d. Begin to urinate while continuing to hold labia apart. Allow first urine to flow into toilet.	
____	____	____	e. Hold specimen container under the urine stream and collect sample.	
____	____	____	f. Remove specimen container, release hand from labia, seal container tightly, and finish voiding; wash hands.	
____	____	____	3. Put on disposable gloves to receive specimen container from the client. Dry outside of container with a paper towel.	
____	____	____	4. Date and time laboratory specimen. Verify the client by two identifiers and make sure they match the label. Label the container and place specimen container in biohazard bag.	
____	____	____	5. Send specimen to laboratory within 15 minutes or place in specimen refrigerator. If specimen is for microbiology testing, it must be sent immediately and not refrigerated.	
____	____	____	6. Dispose of all contaminated supplies. Wash hands.	
			Self-Collecting Midstream Urine Specimen for a Man	
____	____	____	1. Confirm the physician's orders and identify the client with at least two identifiers.	
____	____	____	2. Give the client the following instructions on how to cleanse urinary meatus and obtain urine specimen: a. Wash hands.	
____	____	____	b. Starting at the top in a circular motion, cleanse end of penis with cotton balls and soap or commercially prepared antiseptic swabs. If man is not circumcised, he should retract his foreskin to expose the urinary meatus before cleansing and throughout specimen collection.	
____	____	____	c. Repeat cleansing three times with three separate cotton balls or antiseptic swabs.	
____	____	____	d. Begin to urinate, allowing first urine to flow into toilet.	

Excellent	Satisfactory	Needs Practice	PROCEDURE 41-1 **Collecting Urine Specimens (*Continued*)** **Goal:** To obtain a noncontaminated urine specimen for routine analysis or culture and sensitivity.	Comments
___	___	___	e. Pass specimen container into urine stream and collect sample.	
___	___	___	f. Remove container, seal tightly, and finish voiding.	
___	___	___	3. Follow Steps 3 to 6 above under "Self-Collecting Midstream Urine Specimen for a Woman."	

Collecting a Specimen From a Child Without Urinary Control

Excellent	Satisfactory	Needs Practice		Comments
___	___	___	1. Confirm the physician's order and identify the client with at least two identifiers.	
___	___	___	2. If parents are present, explain procedure to them.	
___	___	___	3. Position child gently on the back. Put on disposable gloves. Remove diaper.	
___	___	___	4. Clean perineal–genital area gently with soap and water, followed by antiseptic.	
___	___	___	5. For a girl: Separate labia and cleanse from front of urethral meatus toward the rectum. Rinse with water and dry with cotton balls.	
___	___	___	6. For a boy: Cleanse the penis and scrotum. If boy is not circumcised, retract the foreskin and cleanse. Rinse with water and dry with gauze or cotton balls.	
___	___	___	7. Remove paper backing from adhesive of collection bag.	
___	___	___	8. Spread the child's legs widely apart.	
___	___	___	9. Apply collection bag over child's perineum, covering penis and scrotum of boy, urinary meatus and vagina of girl. Press adhesive to secure, starting at the perineum and working outward.	
___	___	___	10. Place a diaper on the child loosely.	
___	___	___	11. Remove gloves and wash hands.	
___	___	___	12. Check the collector for urine every 15 minutes. Parents can check child for urine specimen.	
___	___	___	13. When urine specimen is obtained, glove again, gently remove collection bag from the skin, and empty urine into specimen container.	
___	___	___	14. Tighten lid, cleanse outside of container if contaminated with urine, and place in plastic biohazard bag for transfer to the laboratory.	
___	___	___	15. Label the container, making sure that client information is correct. Record date and time on laboratory requisition form.	
___	___	___	16. Send specimen to laboratory within 15 minutes or place in specimen refrigerator. If specimen is for microbiology testing, it must be sent immediately and not refrigerated.	
___	___	___	17. Dispose of all contaminated supplies. Wash hands.	
___	___	___	18. Document that specimen was collected and sent.	

Procedure Checklists for Craven and Hirnle's Fundamentals of Nursing: Human Health and Function, 6th edition

Name _____   Date _____

Unit _____   Position _____

Instructor/Evaluator: _____   Position _____

Excellent	Satisfactory	Needs Practice	PROCEDURE 41-2 **Assessing Urine Volume Using a Bladder Ultrasonic Scanner (BUS)** **Goal:** To noninvasively calculate the volume of urine in the bladder; to determine the need for catheterization to relieve urinary retention.	Comments
____	____	____	1. Identify the client and explain the procedure.	
____	____	____	2. Wash hands. Put on disposable gloves.	
____	____	____	3. Provide privacy; close curtains around bed and close door to room if possible.	
____	____	____	4. Raise the bed to a comfortable working height. Assist the client to lie as flat as can be tolerated comfortably. Expose only the client's lower abdomen and suprapubic area.	
____	____	____	5. Clean scan head probe (soundwave transducer) with isopropyl alcohol.	
____	____	____	6. Turn the bladder scanner on and press scan.	
____	____	____	7. Press *male* or *female* mode on scan device. If a female client has had a hysterectomy (removal of uterus), press *male*.	
____	____	____	8. Gently palpate the client's symphysis pubis, and then apply ultrasound gel midline on the abdomen (about 1 to 1.5 inches above the symphysis pubis). Or apply ultrasound gel directly to the scan head.	
____	____	____	9. Find the symphysis pubis (midline below the umbilicus) and place the scan head approximately 3 cm superior to the symphysis pubis, pointing toward the expected bladder location. Locate the icon on the scan head and point the icon toward the client's head.	
____	____	____	10. Press the scan head button and hold the scan head steady until a beep is heard, then release.	
____	____	____	11. The bladder scan will display the bladder volume measurement and an aiming display. Adjust scan head aim to obtain intersection of the crosshair and the bladder. Reposition the scan head and repeat the measurement as needed to obtain a centered image.	
____	____	____	12. When finished, press done and print for a hard copy of results.	
____	____	____	13. Wipe gel from client's skin and reposition client if needed.	
____	____	____	14. Dispose of contaminated supplies. Clean scan head with isopropyl alcohol. Wash hands.	

Procedure Checklists for Craven and Hirnle's Fundamentals
of Nursing: Human Health and Function, 6th edition

Name _____ Date _____

Unit _____ Position _____

Instructor/Evaluator: _____ Position _____

PROCEDURE 41-3

Applying a Condom Catheter

Goal: To provide a means of collecting urine and controlling incontinence without the risk of infection that an indwelling urinary catheter imposes.

Excellent	Satisfactory	Needs Practice		Comments
____	____	____	1. Close room door or bedside curtain. Explain procedure to client.	
____	____	____	2. Wash hands.	
____	____	____	3. Raise the head of the bed to a comfortable working height. Assist client to supine position with thighs slightly apart. Drape client so that only the area around the genitalia is exposed.	
____	____	____	4. Put on disposable gloves. Wash client's genitals with soap and water. Clean the tip of the penis first using a circular motion from the meatus outward. Wash the shaft of the penis using downward strokes toward the pubic area. Towel dry. For an uncircumcised male, retract the foreskin and clean the glans of the penis. Be sure to replace the foreskin after cleansing.	
____	____	____	5. Trim excess pubic hair from base of penis, if necessary.	
____	____	____	6. Apply thin film of skin protector on penis shaft (usually found in commercially packaged condom catheter kits). Allow to dry for 30 seconds.	
____	____	____	7. Grasp penis firmly with nondominant hand. Apply condom sheath by unrolling the sheath the length of the penis using dominant hand. Leave 1 to 2 inches (2.5–5 cm) of space between the tip of the penis and the end of the condom sheath. Some brands of condom catheters are held in place with a Velcro strap over the condom catheter.	
____	____	____	8. Attach funnel end of condom to collection system tubing. Avoid kinks or loops in the tubing. Secure drainage tubing to client's inner thigh with Velcro leg strap or tape.	
____	____	____	9. Discard used supplies and wash hands.	
____	____	____	10. Assist client to a comfortable position and cover him with bed linens. Place the bed in the lowest position.	

PROCEDURE 41-3
Applying a Condom Catheter (*Continued*)

Excellent	Satisfactory	Needs Practice	**Goal:** To provide a means of collecting urine and controlling incontinence without the risk of infection that an indwelling urinary catheter imposes.	**Comments**
____	____	____	11. Secure collection system bag below the level of the bladder. Check that the tubing is not kinked and that movement of bed rails does not interfere with the drainage system.	
____	____	____	12. Observe penis, 15 to 30 minutes after application of condom, for swelling or changes in skin color. Routinely remove condom, examine the underlying skin, and reapply at least every 24 hours or if client complains of any discomfort.	

*Procedure Checklists for Craven and Hirnle's Fundamentals
of Nursing: Human Health and Function,* 6th edition

Name _____ Date _____

Unit _____ Position _____

Instructor/Evaluator: _____ Position _____

PROCEDURE 41-4
Inserting a Straight or Indwelling Urinary Catheter

Indwelling Catheterization
Goal: To monitor urinary function; to prevent or relieve bladder distention; to provide continuous bladder drainage; to provide a means for irrigating the bladder with fluids or medication.

Straight Catheterization
Goal: To obtain sterile urine specimens; to measure residual urine

Excellent	Satisfactory	Needs Practice		Comments
			Initial Steps for Inserting Straight or Indwelling Catheters	
___	___	___	1. Verify the physician's orders and identify the client. Determine if client has any allergies (especially to iodine and latex).	
___	___	___	2. Explain the procedure and rationale to client. Close curtain around bed and close door to room if possible.	
___	___	___	3. Set up good light source. Place trash receptacle within easy reach.	
___	___	___	4. Raise the bed to a comfortable working height. Stand on the client's right side if you are right-handed, on the client's left side if you are left-handed.	
___	___	___	5. Provide the client with opportunity to perform personal perineal/penile hygiene. If the client is unable or unwilling to perform personal hygiene, assist or perform hygiene as necessary. Perform hand hygiene and put on clean gloves. Slide waterproof pad under client. For the female client, wipe from front to back. For the male client, clean the tip of the penis first, using circular motions from the meatus outward, and then cleanse the shaft of the penis using downward strokes toward the pubic area. Remove gloves and wash hands.	
			Inserting Indwelling Catheter in a Female Client	
___	___	___	1. Position client in dorsal recumbent position (supine with knees flexed). Externally rotate thighs. Side-lying is an alternative position.	
___	___	___	2. Open the catheterization tray on clean bedside table while maintaining asepsis. See Procedure 27-5. If necessary, put on clean gloves. Pick up drape from	

PROCEDURE 41-4
Inserting a Straight or Indwelling Urinary Catheter
(*Continued*)

Excellent	Satisfactory	Needs Practice	**Indwelling Catheterization** **Goal:** To monitor urinary function; to prevent or relieve bladder distention; to provide continuous bladder drainage; to provide a means for irrigating the bladder with fluids or medication. **Straight Catheterization** **Goal:** To obtain sterile urine specimens; to measure residual urine	Comments
			the top of the catheterization kit, touching only the corners of the drape. Slide sterile drape under client's buttocks; ask client to lift hips if possible so drape can be slid under easily. Do not touch center of drape.	
___	___	___	3. If used, remove clean gloves. Don sterile gloves. Place fenestrated sterile drape over the perineal area. Place sterile catheterization tray on sterile drape between client's thighs.	
___	___	___	4. Open sterile lubricant and lubricate the catheter tip. With a physician's order, 2% lidocaine gel can also be used for lubrication. Open cleansing solution and pour over half of the sterile balls or open antimicrobial cleansing swabs. Open the sterile specimen container. Test the catheter balloon by inserting the prefilled sterile water syringe into the injection port and injecting the appropriate amount of fluid. If balloon inflates properly, aspirate fluid back into syringe and leave it attached to the injection port.	
___	___	___	5. Place nondominant hand on labia minora and gently spread to expose urinary meatus. (This hand is now considered contaminated.) Visualize exact location of meatus. During cleansing and catheter insertion, do not allow labia to close over meatus until after the catheter is inserted.	
___	___	___	6. Using sterile hand, pick up saturated cotton ball with sterile forceps or antimicrobial swabs.	
___	___	___	7. Cleanse the urinary meatus with one downward stroke. Discard the cotton ball or antimicrobial swab. Repeat this step three or four times.	
___	___	___	8. Use dry cotton balls to absorb excess antiseptic solution.	
___	___	___	9. With sterile hand, pick up the catheter approximately 3 inches from the tip and place distal catheter end into sterile basin. If the catheter is attached to sterile tubing and drainage container (closed drainage system), position catheter and setup within easy reach on the sterile field. Make sure clamp on drainage bag is closed.	

PROCEDURE 41-4
Inserting a Straight or Indwelling Urinary Catheter
(*Continued*)

Indwelling Catheterization
Goal: To monitor urinary function; to prevent or relieve bladder distention; to provide continuous bladder drainage; to provide a means for irrigating the bladder with fluids or medication.

Straight Catheterization
Goal: To obtain sterile urine specimens; to measure residual urine

Excellent	Satisfactory	Needs Practice		Comments
___	___	___	10. Gently insert catheter into urethra (approximately 2 inches) until urine begins to drain. If no urine appears, have client cough or reposition catheter by rotating. Have client take slow, deep breaths during catheter insertion.	
___	___	___	11. Insert the catheter an additional 1 inch (2.5 cm).	
___	___	___	12. Inflate the retention balloon with the prefilled syringe. Check to ensure placement by gently pulling on catheter.	
___	___	___	13. Connect distal end of catheter to drainage bag. In some kits, the catheter is already connected to the drainage unit. Some nurses prefer to connect equipment before catheter insertion.	
___	___	___	14. Secure catheter tubing to the client's inner thigh with Velcro leg strap or 1-inch tape, with enough give so it will not pull when the legs move.	
___	___	___	15. Attach drainage bag to bed frame, ensuring that tubing does not fall into dependent loops and that side rails do not interfere with drainage system.	
___	___	___	16. Remove gloves and wash hands.	
___	___	___	17. Record the time of completion of the procedure, size of catheter inserted, amount and color of urine, and any adverse client responses.	

Inserting Straight Catheter in a Female Client

___	___	___	1. Follow "Initial Steps for Inserting Straight or Indwelling Catheters."	
___	___	___	2. Follow Steps 1 through 10 of "Inserting Indwelling Catheter in a Female Client."	
___	___	___	3. With sterile hand, place the drainage end of the catheter in a receptacle. If a specimen is required, place the end into the specimen container in the receptacle.	
___	___	___	4. Gently insert catheter into urethra (approximately 2 inches) until urine begins to drain. If no urine appears, have client cough or reposition catheter by rotating. Have client take slow, deep breaths during catheter insertion.	

PROCEDURE 41-4
Inserting a Straight or Indwelling Urinary Catheter
(*Continued*)

Excellent	Satisfactory	Needs Practice	**Indwelling Catheterization** **Goal:** To monitor urinary function; to prevent or relieve bladder distention; to provide continuous bladder drainage; to provide a means for irrigating the bladder with fluids or medication. **Straight Catheterization** **Goal:** To obtain sterile urine specimens; to measure residual urine	**Comments**
___	___	___	5. Hold the catheter securely at the urinary meatus while the bladder empties. If ordered, obtain urine specimen in sterile container, pinching catheter once specimen is obtained. Add volume of specimen to the residual volume obtained.	
___	___	___	6. Allow the bladder to empty completely. Withdraw the catheter slowly and smoothly. Wash and dry genital area as necessary.	
___	___	___	7. Remove gloves and assist client to a comfortable position. Cover the client with a gown and bed linens.	
___	___	___	8. Put on clean gloves. Cover and label urine specimen if applicable and place in plastic bag with lab requisition form. Check client identity with two separate identifiers. Send urine specimen to the laboratory immediately.	
___	___	___	9. Remove gloves and wash hands.	
			Inserting Indwelling Catheter in a Male Client	
___	___	___	1. Position client in supine position with only genitalia exposed.	
___	___	___	2. Drape legs to midthigh with bath blanket or sheet.	
___	___	___	3. Open the sterile catheterization tray on a clean bedside table, maintaining asepsis.	
___	___	___	4. Put on sterile gloves. Place the fenestrated drape over the client's genitalia. Place sterile catheterization tray between client's legs on the sterile drape.	
___	___	___	5. Open cleansing solution and pour over half of the sterile cotton balls, or open antimicrobial swabs. Open the sterile specimen container. To test the catheter balloon, insert the prefilled sterile water syringe into the injection port. Inject the appropriate amount of fluid to inflate the balloon. If balloon inflates properly, aspirate fluid back into syringe and leave attached to the injection port.	
___	___	___	6. Using sterile hand, place the distal catheter end into sterile basin. If catheter is preattached to sterile tubing and drainage container (closed drainage system), position catheter and setup within easy reach on sterile field. Ensure that clamp on drainage	

PROCEDURE 41-4

Inserting a Straight or Indwelling Urinary Catheter
(*Continued*)

Excellent	Satisfactory	Needs Practice	**Indwelling Catheterization** **Goal:** To monitor urinary function; to prevent or relieve bladder distention; to provide continuous bladder drainage; to provide a means for irrigating the bladder with fluids or medication. **Straight Catheterization** **Goal:** To obtain sterile urine specimens; to measure residual urine	Comments
			bag is closed. Remove cap from syringe prefilled with lubricant and squirt onto sterile field.	
____	____	____	7. With your nondominant hand, hold the penis at a 90-degree angle to the body. If the client is not circumcised, pull back the foreskin with this hand to visualize the urethral meatus. (This hand is now considered unsterile.)	
____	____	____	8. Using the sterile hand, pick up the cleansing solution—either antimicrobial swabs or the soaked cotton ball (using sterile forceps).	
____	____	____	9. Cleanse the urinary meatus with one downward stroke or use a circular motion from meatus to base of penis. Discard the cotton ball or antimicrobial swabs. Repeat this step at least three or four times.	
____	____	____	10. Use forceps to pick up one dry cotton ball to dry the meatus.	
____	____	____	11. Hold penis with slight upward tension and perpendicular to the client's body. Lubricate catheter well with lubricant or lidocaine. For a client needing extra lubrication, the lubricant or lidocaine can be injected directly into the penis.	
____	____	____	12. Gently insert catheter into urethra (approximately 8 inches) until urine begins to drain.	
____	____	____	13. Insert catheter an additional 1 inch (2.5 cm).	
____	____	____	14. Inflate the balloon with the prefilled syringe.	
____	____	____	15. Check for placement by gently pulling on catheter.	
____	____	____	16. Connect distal end of catheter to drainage bag if necessary.	
____	____	____	17. Secure catheter tubing to the client's thigh or abdomen using a Velcro leg strap or 1-inch tape. Leave some slack in catheter tubing to allow for movement.	
____	____	____	18. In the uncircumcised male, gently replace the foreskin over the glans.	
____	____	____	19. Attach drainage bag to bed frame, coiling tubing to ensure that tubing does not fall into dependent loops.	
____	____	____	20. Wash hands.	
____	____	____	21. Record the time of completion of the procedure, size of catheter, amount and color of urine, and any adverse client responses.	

PROCEDURE 41-4
Inserting a Straight or Indwelling Urinary Catheter (*Continued*)

Excellent	Satisfactory	Needs Practice	**Indwelling Catheterization** **Goal:** To monitor urinary function; to prevent or relieve bladder distention; to provide continuous bladder drainage; to provide a means for irrigating the bladder with fluids or medication. **Straight Catheterization** **Goal:** To obtain sterile urine specimens; to measure residual urine	**Comments**
			Inserting Straight Catheter in a Male Client	
___	___	___	1. Follow Steps 1 through 5 in "Initial Steps for Inserting Straight or Indwelling Catheters."	
___	___	___	2. Follow Steps 1 through 11 for "Inserting an Indwelling Catheter in a Male Client."	
___	___	___	3. Using your sterile hand, place the drainage end of the catheter in a receptacle. If a specimen is required, place the end into the specimen container in the receptacle.	
___	___	___	4. Gently insert catheter into urethra (approximately 8 inches) until urine begins to drain.	
___	___	___	5. Hold the catheter securely at the meatus with your nondominant hand while the bladder empties. If a specimen is being collected, remove the drainage end of the tubing from the specimen container after the required amount is obtained and allow urine to flow into receptacle. Set specimen container aside.	
___	___	___	6. Allow the bladder to empty completely. Withdraw the catheter slowly and smoothly. Wash and dry genital area as necessary. If necessary, replace foreskin.	
___	___	___	7. Remove gloves and assist client to a comfortable position. Cover the client with a gown and bed linens.	
___	___	___	8. Put on clean gloves. Cover and label urine specimen and place in plastic bag with lab requisition form. Check client identity with two separate identifiers. Send urine specimen to the laboratory immediately.	
___	___	___	9. Remove gloves and wash hands.	
			Removing an Indwelling Catheter	
___	___	___	1. Identify the client. Explain the procedure.	
___	___	___	2. Wash your hands. Don clean, disposable gloves.	
___	___	___	3. Close curtains around bed and close door to room if possible.	
___	___	___	4. Position client as for catheter insertion. Drape client so that only the area around the catheter is exposed. Place a waterproof pad under the female client's legs or over the male client's thighs.	
___	___	___	5. Clamp the catheter (optional).	

PROCEDURE 41-4

Inserting a Straight or Indwelling Urinary Catheter (*Continued*)

Indwelling Catheterization
Goal: To monitor urinary function; to prevent or relieve bladder distention; to provide continuous bladder drainage; to provide a means for irrigating the bladder with fluids or medication.

Straight Catheterization
Goal: To obtain sterile urine specimens; to measure residual urine

Excellent	Satisfactory	Needs Practice		Comments
____	____	____	6. Remove the Velcro leg strap or tape used to secure the catheter tubing to the client's thigh or abdomen.	
____	____	____	7. Insert hub of syringe into balloon inflation tube of catheter and draw out all liquid. Size of balloon is indicated on catheter; most commonly, sizes smaller than 10 mL are used. Larger balloons (30 mL) may be used after prostatic or urologic surgery.	
____	____	____	8. Ask client to breathe in and out deeply. Pinch catheter and remove slowly and gently as client exhales.	
____	____	____	9. Place catheter on waterproof pad and wrap in pad.	
____	____	____	10. Assist client to cleanse and dry genitals. Remove gloves and assist client to a comfortable position. Place gown over client and cover the client with bed linens.	
____	____	____	11. Put on clean gloves. Remove and dispose of used equipment according to agency policy. Measure and document urine in drainage bag and time of catheter removal. Estimate when client should void (within 8 hours).	
____	____	____	12. Remove gloves and wash hands.	

Procedure Checklists for Craven and Hirnle's Fundamentals
of Nursing: Human Health and Function, 6th edition

Name _____ Date _____

Unit _____ Position _____

Instructor/Evaluator: _____ Position _____

Excellent	Satisfactory	Needs Practice	PROCEDURE 42-1 **Assessing Stool for Occult Blood**	Comments
			Goal: To screen clients who have or who are at risk for gastrointestinal bleeding; to screen for early-stage colon cancer.	
___	___	___	1. Identify client. Ask the client to void before collecting the stool specimen.	
___	___	___	2. Assist client onto bedpan or commode or to bathroom. Provide privacy; leave call bell handy.	
___	___	___	3. Once the client has passed stool and is clean and comfortable, don disposable gloves and obtain small amount of stool with a tongue blade or wooden applicator.	
			Hemoccult Slide Test	
___	___	___	1. Open flap of slide and apply a very thin smear of stool taken from the center of the specimen onto first window.	
___	___	___	2. Using second applicator, obtain a second sample from a different area of the stool. Smear thinly on second window of slide.	
___	___	___	3. Close slide cover. Wait 3 to 5 minutes; then open flap on reverse side and apply two drops of Hemoccult developing solution onto each window and one drop onto control window.	
___	___	___	4. Wait 30 to 60 seconds. Read test results. 5. Remove gloves, wash hands, and document findings.	

Procedure Checklists for Craven and Hirnle's Fundamentals of Nursing: Human Health and Function, 6th edition

Name _____ Date _____

Unit _____ Position _____

Instructor/Evaluator: _____ Position _____

PROCEDURE 42-2
Administering an Enema

Goal: To relieve gas, constipation, or fecal impaction; to cleanse the bowel in preparation for diagnostic tests or surgical procedures; to evacuate feces in clients with hemiplegia, quadriplegia, or paraplegia; to deliver medication.

Excellent	Satisfactory	Needs Practice		Comments
			Large-Volume Enema	
___	___	___	1. Assemble the needed equipment in one place.	
___	___	___	2. Prepare solution. Check temperature of solution by pouring some over your inner wrist. Fill enema bag with 750 to 1000 mL lukewarm solution (105° to 110°F; for child, 500 mL or less, 100°F).	
___	___	___	3. Open clamp on tubing and allow solution to flow through tubing to remove the air. Reclamp tubing.	
___	___	___	4. Provide privacy by closing curtains or room door.	
___	___	___	5. Identify client. Position client on left side (Sims' position) with right knee flexed.	
___	___	___	6. Cover client with bath blanket, exposing only the rectum.	
___	___	___	7. Put on disposable gloves. Place waterproof pad under client's buttocks.	
___	___	___	8. Lubricate 2 to 3 inches of the tip of the rectal tube with water-soluble lubricant.	
___	___	___	9. Separate the buttocks to visualize the anus. Observe for external hemorrhoids. Ask client to take a slow, deep breath. Gently insert the tube, directing the tip toward the umbilicus (adult: 3–4 inches).	
___	___	___	10. Continue holding the tube in the rectum. With other hand, open the clamp and allow solution to slowly enter the client. Raise container 18 inches above the anus, allowing solution to flow slowly over 5 to 10 minutes. If client complains of cramping or pain, have client breathe deeply and lower bag until the sensation stops.	
___	___	___	11. Reclamp tubing when desired amount of solution has infused.	
___	___	___	12. Remove tube gently and have client squeeze buttocks together firmly for several minutes.	
___	___	___	13. Have client retain solution as long as possible.	
___	___	___	14. Assist client to bathroom, commode, or bedpan. Place call bell within reach. Provide privacy until all of the solution has been expelled.	
___	___	___	15. Visually inspect character of the feces and solution.	

PROCEDURE 42-2
Administering an Enema (*Continued*)

Excellent	Satisfactory	Needs Practice	**Goal:** To relieve gas, constipation, or fecal impaction; to cleanse the bowel in preparation for diagnostic tests or surgical procedures; to evacuate feces in clients with hemiplegia, quadriplegia, or paraplegia; to deliver medication.	Comments
___	___	___	16. Assist client into comfortable position. Assist with cleansing as needed. Provide materials for client to wash hands. Open windows or provide air freshener if needed. Clean and dispose of equipment as necessary. Remove gloves and wash hands.	
			Small-Volume Enema	
___	___	___	1. Assemble the needed equipment in one place.	
___	___	___	2. Provide privacy by closing curtains or room door.	
___	___	___	3. Identify client. Position client on left side (Sims' position) with right knee flexed.	
___	___	___	4. Put on disposable gloves. Place waterproof towel under client's buttocks.	
___	___	___	5. Cover client with bath blanket, exposing only the rectum.	
___	___	___	6. Remove protective cap from prelubricated catheter tip. You may add more lubricant if necessary.	
___	___	___	7. Separate the buttocks to visualize the anus. Observe for hemorrhoids and gently insert rectal tip into rectum, directing the tip toward the umbilicus.	
___	___	___	8. Squeeze bottle to empty contents into the rectum and colon (approximately 240 mL of solution).	
___	___	___	9. Maintain pressure on the enema container until you withdraw it from the rectum.	
___	___	___	10. Continue with steps 13–16 above for a large-volume enema.	

Procedure Checklists for Craven and Hirnle's Fundamentals of Nursing: Human Health and Function, 6th edition

Name _____   Date _____

Unit _____   Position _____

Instructor/Evaluator: _____   Position _____

PROCEDURE 42-3
Inserting a Nasogastric Tube

Goal: To decompress the stomach to relieve pressure and prevent vomiting; to provide a means for irrigating the stomach (lavage); to provide access to gastric specimens for laboratory analysis; to provide a route for delivering liquid enteral feedings (gavage) in clients who can't swallow or ingest adequate calorie intake (see Chapter 38).

Excellent	Satisfactory	Needs Practice		Comments
____	____	____	1. Identify client and explain procedure. Insertion is not painful, but it is uncomfortable because the gag reflex is usually stimulated.	
____	____	____	2. Provide privacy by closing curtains or room door. Raise bed to high-Fowler's position, cover chest with towel or drape, and place emesis basin nearby.	
____	____	____	3. Wash hands, and put on gloves. Determine length of tubing to be inserted by measuring nasogastric tube from tip of earlobe to tip of nose, then to tip of xiphoid process. Mark tubing with adhesive tape or note striped markings already on the tube.	
____	____	____	4. Lubricate tip of tube with water-soluble lubricant.	
____	____	____	5. Gently insert tube into nostril. Advance toward posterior pharynx.	
____	____	____	6. Have client tilt head forward and encourage client to drink water slowly. Advance tube without using force as client swallows. Advance tube until desired insertion length is reached.	
____	____	____	7. Temporarily tape the tube to the client's nose; then assess placement of the tube:	
____	____	____	a. Aspirate gastric content with 20- to 50-mL syringe; note color and test pH. If the pH is ≤5, it can be assumed that the tube is in the stomach.	
____	____	____	b. Although not supported by current evidence, some nurses carefully inject 10 to 20 mL air into the nasogastric tube while auscultating over the epigastrium.	
____	____	____	c. If feeding tube is placed, x-ray confirmation of placement is required before feeding is administered.	
____	____	____	8. If placement in stomach is not correct, untape tube, advance tube 5 cm, and repeat assessment in Step 7.	
____	____	____	9. Secure tube by taping to bridge of client's nose. Anchor tubing to client's gown.	
____	____	____	10. Clamp end of tubing or attach to suction, as ordered by healthcare provider.	

PROCEDURE 42-3
Inserting a Nasogastric Tube (*Continued*)

Excellent	Satisfactory	Needs Practice	**Goal:** To decompress the stomach to relieve pressure and prevent vomiting; to provide a means for irrigating the stomach (lavage); to provide access to gastric specimens for laboratory analysis; to provide a route for delivering liquid enteral feedings (gavage) in clients who can't swallow or ingest adequate calorie intake (see Chapter 38).	**Comments**
____	____	____	11. Wash hands, provide for client's comfort, and remove equipment.	
____	____	____	12. Establish and document a plan for daily care of the nasogastric tube:	
____	____	____	a. Inspect nostril for irritation.	
____	____	____	b. Cleanse nostril frequently.	
____	____	____	c. Change adhesive as required to prevent skin irritation or pressure sores on nostril from the tube.	
____	____	____	d. Increase frequency of oral care because clients with nasogastric tubes often mouth breathe and may be NPO.	

Procedure Checklists for Craven and Hirnle's Fundamentals of Nursing: Human Health and Function, 6th edition

Name _____   Date _____

Unit _____   Position _____

Instructor/Evaluator: _____   Position _____

PROCEDURE 42-4
Applying a Fecal Ostomy Pouch

Goal: To contain drainage and odors for the comfort of the client and allows accurate assessment of output; to protect the peristomal skin from excoriation; to allow accurate assessment of output, especially in the postoperative period; to provide visualization of the stoma and sutures during the postoperative period.

Excellent	Satisfactory	Needs Practice		Comments
___	___	___	1. Identify client and provide privacy. Don disposable gloves. The client may perform the procedure without gloves. Place a waterproof pad by stoma site.	
___	___	___	2. Gently remove old appliance (and skin barrier if applicable) by pushing skin away from appliance (do not pull appliance from skin); start at the top of the appliance. If disposable, discard. If reusable, set aside for washing.	
___	___	___	3. Use toilet tissue to remove excess stool. Wash skin thoroughly around stoma with skin cleanser or soap and water.	
___	___	___	4. Rinse skin thoroughly and blot dry.	
___	___	___	5. Observe condition of peristomal skin, the stoma, and the sutures. Teach the client to make these observations daily.	
___	___	___	6. Cover stoma with gauze while you prepare new appliance. Prepare appliance and/or skin barrier: measure stoma using a measurement guide and trace stoma measurement on the adhesive paper backing of appliance or barrier. Cut the opening ⅛ inch larger than tracing.	
___	___	___	7. If stoma is located in an abdominal crease or the skin is irregular, use a paste barrier to fill the irregularity.	
___	___	___	8. Apply protectant as needed/desired. Allow protectant to dry completely.	
___	___	___	9. Apply protective skin barrier.	
___	___	___	a. Peel paper backing off wafer, and center stoma in hole.	
___	___	___	b. Place on abdomen, pressing lightly over all areas of the barrier to promote adhesion with skin surfaces.	

PROCEDURE 42-4
Applying a Fecal Ostomy Pouch (*Continued*)

Excellent	Satisfactory	Needs Practice	**Goal:** To contain drainage and odors for the comfort of the client and allows accurate assessment of output; to protect the peristomal skin from excoriation; to allow accurate assessment of output, especially in the postoperative period; to provide visualization of the stoma and sutures during the postoperative period.	**Comments**
___	___	___	10. Attach drainable pouch to skin barrier. Some equipment attaches by means of a plastic flange that snaps in place; other models adhere through self-adherent tape that is exposed after protective paper backing is removed. Tug gently or inspect for secure fit.	
___	___	___	11. Fold over bottom edge of pouch and clamp.	
___	___	___	12. Dispose of old appliance. Clean and store any reusable supplies. Wash hands. Document observations.	

Procedure Checklists for Craven and Hirnle's Fundamentals of Nursing: Human Health and Function, 6th edition

Name _____ Date _____

Unit _____ Position _____

Instructor/Evaluator: _____ Position _____

Excellent	Satisfactory	Needs Practice	PROCEDURE 44-1 **Pain Management: Epidural Analgesia**	Comments
			Goal: To administer medications via a patient-controlled epidural analgesia system.	
___	___	___	1. Check physician order for current analgesia dose.	
___	___	___	2. Wash hands.	
___	___	___	3. Place epidural safety sign over head of bed.	
___	___	___	4. Insert tubing into medication bag; prime tubing and filter. Place tubing in pump with proper rate set to deliver ordered dose. Set limit to the amount of fluid in bag. Place epidural catheter label on tubing near pump.	
___	___	___	5. Cleanse connector of epidural catheter with antiseptic swab. Wipe dry with sterile gauze.	
___	___	___	6. Remove cap from epidural catheter. Attach 3-mL syringe and aspirate. Moderate resistance will be felt. If more than 0.5 mL clear fluid or any blood is aspirated, *stop aspiration.* Remove syringe, recap catheter. Do not inject any fluid into catheter. Notify the anesthesia department immediately.	
___	___	___	7. If less than 0.5 mL fluid is aspirated, remove syringe and connect tubing and filter to the client's epidural catheter. Confirm that all connections are secure. Confirm that epidural catheter label is in place on epidural catheter.	
___	___	___	8. Recheck pump settings against physician's orders and turn on pump. Many agencies consider this a high-risk medication and require two nurses to double-check each other when the epidural infusion is started or changed.	
___	___	___	9. Follow medical orders for ongoing monitoring of pain level, vital signs, and sensory-motor function.	

*Procedure Checklists for Craven and Hirnle's Fundamentals
of Nursing: Human Health and Function,* 6th edition

Name _____ Date _____

Unit _____ Position _____

Instructor/Evaluator: _____ Position _____

PROCEDURE 44-2
Pain Management: Patient-Controlled Analgesia

Goal: To allow a client to safely self-administer small preset doses of prescribed analgesic intravenously; with continuous infusion, to allow a client to receive a baseline continuous IV infusion of analgesic and also to safely self-administer small preset doses of prescribed analgesic as needed for increased pain.

Excellent	Satisfactory	Needs Practice		Comments

Initiating PCA Therapy

1. Explain PCA to the client.
   a. Explain to visitors/family that only the client is to use the "pain button." *Visitors/family may not push the "pain button" for the client.*
   b. Reinforce teaching throughout course of therapy.
   c. Document client and family teaching.
2. Check the label on the prefilled syringe with the medication record and the client's identification. Some agencies require two nurses to double-check this.
3. Connect prefilled syringe to the PCA device tubing. Load syringe into PCA device.
4. Prime PCA device tubing. Program infusion dose and lockout interval according to the medical order.
5. Lock PCA device and remove key.
6. Clean port with antimicrobial swab. Connect the PCA device tubing to the client's primary IV tubing. Activate PCA device by pressing the start button.
7. Instruct client to press button when experiencing pain. Reassure client that lockout prevents possible overdose.
8. Document administration of medication immediately, including date, time, dose, lockout interval, and any other observations of IV site and primary IV infusion.

Monitoring and Discontinuing PCA Therapy

1. Check the IV site frequently for signs of infiltration or occlusion.
2. If a client is no longer capable of administering his or her medications, notify the physician so that another method of pain management can be used.

PROCEDURE 44-2

Pain Management: Patient-Controlled Analgesia
(*Continued*)

Excellent	Satisfactory	Needs Practice	**Goal:** To allow a client to safely self-administer small preset doses of prescribed analgesic intravenously; with continuous infusion, to allow a client to receive a baseline continuous IV infusion of analgesic and also to safely self-administer small preset doses of prescribed analgesic as needed for increased pain.	Comments
⎯⎯	⎯⎯	⎯⎯	3. If problems occur, refer to the troubleshooting guide on the pump. The pain management nurse specialist and IV team also can help with problems related to PCA.	
⎯⎯	⎯⎯	⎯⎯	4. A physician's order is required for discontinuation of the PCA. The infusion may be stopped but not discontinued and oral pain medications given.	
⎯⎯	⎯⎯	⎯⎯	5. Discard medication remaining in a syringe. Record action on computerized narcotic distribution cart. Another nurse must witness and enter into the record *wasted* drug.	
⎯⎯	⎯⎯	⎯⎯	6. Record total medication dose (mg/mcg), milliliters (mL) infused, and milliliters (mL) left in the client's record *every shift*.	
⎯⎯	⎯⎯	⎯⎯	7. Document times of syringe changes on the medication administration record (MAR).	

Procedure Checklists for Craven and Hirnle's Fundamentals of Nursing: Human Health and Function, 6th edition

Name _____   Date _____

Unit _____   Position _____

Instructor/Evaluator: _____   Position _____

Excellent	Satisfactory	Needs Practice	PROCEDURE 45-1 **Removing Contact Lenses**	Comments
			Goal: To remove contact lenses in the event that the client is unable to do so.	
			Removing Hard Contact Lenses	
___	___	___	1. Wash hands with soap and warm water.	
___	___	___	2. Position client comfortably in a sitting position, if possible.	
___	___	___	3. Pull the client's upper and lower lid apart and pull tautly toward the lateral side.	
___	___	___	4. Ask the client to blink and the lens should pop out into your hand.	
___	___	___	5. An alternative method for removing hard contact lenses is the use of a lens suction cup. This is particularly useful for a client who cannot consciously assist with the removal.	
			Removing Soft Contact Lenses	
___	___	___	1. Wash hands with soap and warm water.	
___	___	___	2. Position client comfortably in a sitting position, if possible.	
___	___	___	3. Ask the client to look upward. Pull down on the lower lid and place your index finger on the lower edge of the lens, moving it onto the white part of the eye.	
___	___	___	4. Gently grasp lens between your thumb and index finger to release the suction of the lens. The lens will fold over and can easily be removed. Gently roll the lens, using normal saline as needed, to separate it and return it to its normal form.	
			Storing Lenses	
___	___	___	1. Rinse lenses thoroughly with recommended rinsing solution.	
___	___	___	2. Identify the left and right cups marked on the storage case.	
___	___	___	3. Place the first lens in its designated cup in the storage case before removing the second lens.	

Procedure Checklists for Craven and Hirnle's Fundamentals
of Nursing: Human Health and Function, 6th edition

Name _____ Date _____

Unit _____ Position _____

Instructor/Evaluator: _____ Position _____

Excellent	Satisfactory	Needs Practice	PROCEDURE 45-2 **Assisting an Adult With Inserting a Hearing Aid** **Goal:** To maintain hearing status; to provide assistance with insertion.	Comments
____	____	____	1. Check to be sure the battery is functional. Hold hearing aid in your hand and turn up the volume until you hear a "feedback" whistle. The feedback results from sound leaking around and back into the microphone and being amplified.	
____	____	____	2. Inspect the hearing aid to be sure that tubing and ear mold are intact and not cracked or broken. The opening in the ear mold should be free of cerumen.	
____	____	____	3. Clean hearing aid according to manufacturer's guidelines. Place in storage unit.	
____	____	____	4. Assess client's ear for redness, irritation, drainage, and excessive cerumen. Moisten swab and clean ear as necessary.	
____	____	____	5. With the volume turned down, insert the ear mold into the ear canal, twisting slightly for a snug fit.	
____	____	____	6. Secure the battery behind the ear, if of that type. There are other styles of hearing aids that may fit in other ways.	
____	____	____	7. Turn the volume up slowly while speaking to the client in a normal voice tone. Ask the client to let you know when the sound level is comfortable.	